Portfolios in the Nursing Profession

Use in assessment and professional development

Portfolios in the Nursing Profession

Use in assessment and professional development

edited by

Kay Norman

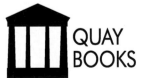

QUAY
BOOKS

Quay Books Division, MA Healthcare Ltd, St Jude's Church, Dulwich Road, London SE24 0PB

British Library Cataloguing-in-Publication Data
A catalogue record is available for this book

© MA Healthcare Limited 2008
ISBN-10: 1-85642-342-5
ISBN-13: 978-1-85642-342-7

Printed in the UK by CLE Print Ltd, Media House, Burell Road, St Ives, PE27 3LE

Contents

List of contributors

Claire Bethell MSc, BA, RHV, RM, RN
Claire is a Principal Lecturer within the Faculty of Health at Staffordshire University and co-ordinates the continuing professional development (undergraduate) scheme, which comprises a wide range of modules and awards. She has an extensive background in health visiting and education within public health. Claire's interest in portfolios began in 1995 when she co-authored a published personal professional portfolio for nurses.

James Dooher MA, FHE Cert Ed, Dip HCR ILTM, RMN
James is a Principal Lecturer and academic lead for mental health within the School of Health and Life Sciences at De Montfort University Leicester. He has worked in a variety of mental health settings and published a number of books, papers and articles related to empowerment, practice development, housing and, most recently, new ways of working in mental health.

Nicky Genders MA, BA(Hons), Cert Ed, RMNH
Nicky is a Principal Lecturer in Nursing within the School of Nursing and Midwifery at De Montfort University Leicester. She has a lead for key skill development having undertaken a number of funded projects over the past five years. She was recently involved in a research project examining key skill development within portfolio-based learning. She has presented both nationally and internationally on employability, key skill development and the nursing portfolio.

Pat Hibberd BEd(Hons), RN, RM, RHV
Pat is a Principal Lecturer for Professional Education at Staffordshire University, a role which includes leadership of mentorship and teacher continuing development. She is currently completing a Doctor of Education programme and has explored the role of portfolio development in continuing professional development.

Val Nixon MSc, BSc(Hons), RN(DiP)
Val is a Senior Lecturer for Emergency/Unscheduled Care in the Faculty of Health at Staffordshire University. Val also has a joint appointment with the West Midlands Strategic Health Authority as a project lead for Emergency Care. Previous work in this role included a project that scoped the Emergency Care nursing workforce. As a result of this project ongoing development of an educational and career framework is currently being undertaken with a view to national implementation.

Kay Norman MSc, PGDHE, BSc(Hons), RGN
Kay is a Principal Lecturer in Primary Health Care within the Faculty of Health at Staffordshire University. She leads on practice nurse education, non-medical prescribing and the development of primary care within pre-registration nursing programmes, and has initiated various modules to include portfolio development as a method of assessment. She also maintains clinical practice working as a contraception and sexual health nurse within Wolverhampton Primary Care Trust on a part-time basis.

Rosemary Shepherd MSc, BSc (Hons), CNT, RGN
Rosemary is a Principal Lecturer within the Faculty of Health at Staffordshire University. Working in close co-operation with academic and trust colleagues within the NHS, Rosemary now takes an operational overview of teaching, learning and assessment for the Health Awards provision within the Faculty. She is also co-ordinator of the accreditation of prior (experiential) learning for the Faculty.

Introduction

Kay Norman

Portfolio development in nursing is continuing to gain momentum both as a strategy for academic assessment and as a method for providing evidence of continuing professional development. A portfolio provides a compilation of evidence relating to your learning journey, which may consist of reflections, testimonials from colleagues/managers, observations, and clinical experiences that are personal to you.

The depth and breadth of this information is dependent on the potential use of the portfolio and will vary according to whether it forms part of an interview process, or must be completed for an academic programme within a higher educational setting. Whatever their use, portfolios are here to stay and should be embraced as a tremendous learning opportunity.

From the editor's and contributing authors' experience both in clinical practice and as educators, it is felt that issues arising from portfolio development continue to be raised by students and qualified nurses, with common queries of, 'I just don't know where to start' and 'What shall I include?' Therefore it is our intention within this text to address some of these issues to help you gain an understanding of the essence of portfolio development in relation to recognising and identifying learning; objective setting and action planning, including information and advice on how to organise your portfolio; types of evidence that may be useful to include; its relation to assessment and lifelong learning; and how this can lead to an enjoyable and empowering process.

Within the various chapters there are examples of templates that you may wish to use for your own portfolio, or to act as a basis for your own ideas and development.

Whatever your reason for developing a portfolio, which is personal to you and your learning, this book will help you to approach its development with enthusiasm and the knowledge that it will be an enjoyable and rewarding learning journey.

Acknowledgements

I gratefully acknowledge the encouragement and contribution of colleagues, family and friends, but most importantly, students in the nursing profession who have provided me and the contributing authors with the essential debate, ideas and issues around portfolio development over a number of years.

I would like to thank those publishers who have given permission to include figures and tables within this book. While every effort has been made to trace all the original copyright holders, if any have inadvertently been overlooked, the publisher will be pleased to make the necessary amendments at the first opportunity.

CHAPTER 1

Facilitating and assessing student learning: Understanding the role of the portfolio

Pat Hibberd

Introduction

In order to understand the role of the portfolio in facilitating and assessing learning, it is important to appreciate its place in the context of changing ideas about knowledge and learning. This chapter gives a brief outline of the educational context in which portfolios are situated, in order that you might have a better understanding of the role and purpose of the portfolio in your course. Once you have an understanding of the context for the portfolio in facilitating and assessing your learning, it will be easier for you to explore and relate to the expectations that undertaking a portfolio in learning and assessment place upon you as a learner. These expectations include the ability to demonstrate the process of learning within the portfolio. This calls for the development of appropriate study skills, the ability to recognise the importance of previous learning and the use of a reflective approach to learning. Finally the chapter introduces the concept of action planning as an important aspect of portfolio planning and development.

The context for portfolios

In the past, professional education was based on the transmission of theoretical knowledge and skills to students who then applied what they had learnt to professional practice (Dall 'Alba, 2004). Freshwater and Stickley (2004) argue that, historically, the transmission of theoretical and practical knowledge in nurse education was heavily influenced by the medical model with ideas and values taken from positivistic science. In this view of learning the student may be seen as a passive receptacle and consequently the responsibility for learning tends to lie with the teacher rather than the learner (Brockbank and McGill, 1998). In recent years however, this transmission model of education has been criticised as being inadequate for professional practice because when theory is generated and taught in one world (eg. in an educational establishment) and then applied by professionals in another (eg. in the world of practice) it can lack relevance or be difficult to apply to practice situations (Schon, 1983, Ghaye and Ghaye, 1998). In addition, it fails to acknowledge that learners have different and individual orientations to learning.

In contrast, it has been argued that practitioners draw on knowledge that has been developed through the experience of professional practice with contemporary professional thinking calling for an interaction between disciplinary knowledge and the implicit knowledge developed by practitioners during their experience of practice (Schon, 1983; Ghaye and Ghaye, 1998; Clarke and Wilcockson, 2001). Experience therefore plays an important role in ideas about how practitioners learn and develop knowledge. For example, when encountering an experience for the first time individuals may be aware of a deficit in knowledge or skill which prevents them from competent practice, this becoming a potential learning experience. Experiential learning may then be gained to meet the deficit in a variety of ways (Jarvis, 2004). A variety of experiential learning strategies may be adopted:

- reading to gain further knowledge and evidence for practice,
- observing another experienced practitioner or mentor,
- asking questions,
- supervised practice,
- clinical supervision,
- role play,
- undertaking a simulated experience,
- reflection in and on action.

In this experiential process learners actively construct their own knowledge based on their ongoing experiences, with learning also subjective to the social and cultural context in which learners find themselves (Jarvis, 2004). These ideas are underpinned by adult learning theory in which the learner is seen as self-motivated and self-directed (Knowles, 1975). However, as Dewar and Walker (1999) identify, supervisory support is also an essential aspect of experiential, work-based learning. Supervisors/mentors in the workplace are important because they can help learners to identify:

- identify the potential learning that the experience can offer,
- identify existing knowledge and relate it to new areas of practice,
- articulate their learning for their portfolio.

In addition, supervisors are vital for public protection ensuring that inexperienced practitioners are supervised while undertaking the necessary experiences that enable them to learn competent practice.

The importance of disciplinary or propositional theory learnt within the classroom and through modes of independent study is of great importance as it forms essential knowledge that must be utilised when the accountable practitioner is deciding how to act in a practice environment (Edwards, 1997). Indeed, Eraut (1992, cited by Taylor, 1997) has identified that professional knowledge includes three types:

- *Propositional knowledge*: the formal, theoretical knowledge developed by and belonging to the discipline or related disciplines.
- *Process knowledge*: this is about knowing how to conduct the different processes which contribute to knowledgeable professional action. This would include the ability to select questions and collect evidence for practice, to problem solve and engage in decision making, to communicate clearly, to self-monitor performance and to manage self in the context of professional practice.
- *Personal knowledge*: this is the ability to understand how personal tacit assumptions and values may be impacting upon decision making processes and delivery of professional practice.

In addition to these forms of knowledge, the concept of emotional intelligence has been highlighted as important for professional practice, including factors such as self-awareness, self-motivation and self-regulation (Cadman and Brewer, 2001).

The changing view of professional knowledge has also given rise to the idea of the 'reflective practitioner', professionals who are able to reflect upon their experiences in order to continually develop their own knowledge. This process is argued to help practitioners cope with working within today's rapidly changing health provision, enabling accountable and appropriate decision making within the new situations constantly presented (Edwards, 1997). Reflection is seen as a mental process applied to complex practice problems for which no obvious solutions are present and is therefore strongly linked to experiential learning. In addition, the outcomes of reflection enable practitioners to engage in a process of building theory from the tacit knowledge gained through practice experiences (Moon, 2004).

Reflection is discussed in more depth in *Chapter 3*.

Continuous learning

The changing nature of professional knowledge has influenced the way that professional education is delivered. A key purpose of any programme of higher education that students undertake will be to facilitate the development of the learning capabilities that enable them to acquire and use these different aspects of professional knowledge. In addition, because the knowledge that underpins professional practice is continually changing it is clear that learning must also be a continuous process and one that is clearly focused on competent practice. This means that developing a disposition to lifelong, work-based, experiential learning will be essential in enabling practitioners to continually improve knowledge and identify and close any skills gaps that impact on the effectiveness and efficiency of practice delivery (Department for Education and Skills, 2003).

Within health and other professions, lifelong learning is often used interchangeably with, or replaced by, the concept of preparing professionals for a lifetime of 'continuing professional development' (CPD). This has been defined as the ongoing individual learning and change that takes place in order to maintain, improve or develop new competence within a professional role (Gopee, 2001). In healthcare policy it is argued that CPD enables the efficient and effective delivery of healthcare priorities and outcomes in order to improve the health economy (UKCC, 1999; Department of Health, 2001) and is seen as an important element in the achievement of government objectives for the NHS (Department of Health, 1999, 2000, 2001).

Being prepared for lifelong learning means that in educational programmes you will be required to demonstrate that you have a number of attributes related to being a lifelong learner, which, according to Crick and Wilson (2005) are:

- *Being self-aware*: knowing what you need to learn in order to update or improve your own performance.
- *Being open and receptive to new learning* and willing to change as a result.
- *Taking responsibility for directing your own learning*: in a professional career you may not have someone to teach what you need to learn.
- *Being able to develop trusting relationships*: we need to be able to work and learn with others in order to cope confidently with uncertainty and change.

Indeed the Dearing Report (National Committee of Inquiry into Higher Education, 1997) included in its recommendations that higher education institutions should implement learning and teaching strategies that focus on the promotion of lifelong learning, self-monitoring and reflection.

These changing ideas about knowledge and adult and experiential learning have therefore been a major factor in the increasing use of portfolios in educational programmes. Neades (2003) argues that the portfolio is a tool that allows learners to structure ongoing development in the light of their own experience, by identifying and recording learning deficits (learning needs) and recording the strategies and actions to be used to address these needs. In addition, the portfolio enables the learner to record and provide evidence of the learning gained as a result of experience, theoretical exploration and reflection, closely integrating theory with practice in so doing (Neades, 2003). Because portfolios are able to record learning over time they are also seen as useful in developing an individual's lifelong learning skills and seen as essential for providing evidence of ongoing professional development for qualified practitioners.

Consequently, in higher educational programmes, portfolios play a key role in facilitating the development of reflective practice and the independent lifelong learner. They also help to identify and equate any gaps in performance with learning needs and direct learning accordingly. These are very important aspects of professional education because they enable professionals to recognise the boundaries of their competence and develop the ability to regulate their own performance.

Assessment of competence

Professionals need to demonstrate, through assessment, the competencies or proficiencies identified by their professional regulatory body, with portfolios being increasingly used as an assessment tool in professional learning and practice (Endacott *et al*, 2004). Although competence can be difficult to define, Gonsci's (1994) holistic model of competence is thought to be helpful (Watson *et al*, 2002; McMullan *et al*, 2003).

Within this holistic view of competence the Department of Health (2006a: 49) has also recently defined competence as the

> *consistent integration of skills, knowledge, attitudes, values and abilities that underpin safe and effective performance in a professional or occupational role.*

These definitions are useful in allowing for the inclusion of different aspects of professional knowledge, abilities and practice into competence and competence assessment (McMullan *et al*, 2003). When using these definitions it should be clear that assessment is not just about the ability to repeat taught propositional disciplinary knowledge as in more traditional approaches to learning, but will include the demonstration of different aspects of personal and process knowledge, such as the ability to problem solve, make decisions, reflect and be self-aware.

Modern competency or proficiency standards reflect these complex and holistic combinations of attributes. As described by Stuart (2003) aspects of professional competence include practitioners being:

- able to use and transfer skills and knowledge across situations,
- up to date,

- self-aware and knowing their limitations,
- able to maintain practice standards identified by professional regulatory body,
- able to recognise abnormalities and take appropriate action,
- able to follow approved policies and procedures,
- in possession of relevant skills for competent practice,
- able to manage contingencies,
- able to teach others,
- able to recognise that competence is context specific.

Because competence is holistic, judgement of competence has to be inferred from a practitioner's performance, and although the assessor's observation of practice plays a central role in judging competence, normally holistic competence cannot be achieved by observation alone. For example, the assessor will need more information about other aspects of practice such as abilities in self-assessment, problem solving and critical thinking processes. Consequently the assessor will need to review other types of evidence in order make a valid and reliable inference of competence and standard of proficiency.

Portfolios are increasingly valued for their use as a tool for recording this range of authentic primary evidence around holistic competence including the provision of evidence and critical commentary on practice (Baume *et al*, 2004). They are increasingly being used in education for both formative (developmental) and summative (final) assessment of specific standards, competencies and learning outcomes (Corcoran and Nicholson, 2004). During the learning and assessment process learners aim to collect and present to their assessors a portfolio that contains a breadth and depth of evidence which demonstrates the range of professional knowledge, skills and attitudes needed for defined standards or competencies (Stuart, 2003). In addition, evidence of portfolio processes such as self-assessment and management of own learning contribute to demonstrating self-monitoring and regulation abilities to maintain knowledge and practice beyond the point of registration in accordance with the requirements of professional self-regulation.

Professional self-regulation

Professional self-regulation is defined by Davis (2000) as where legal recognition is gained by a profession for:

- establishing a register of its qualified practitioners,
- making decisions on the appropriate initial education leading to defined codes and standards for practice,
- restricting registration and practice to those practising within those recognised codes and standards of practice.

The aim of such self-regulation, it has been argued, is to increase the trust given to professionals by a risk aware general public, assuring them that professionals can be expected to act in a certain way (Frowe, 2005). An important part of professional self-regulation is the duty that practitioners have in ensuring that they maintain and work within the boundaries of their professional knowledge and competence and demonstrate this throughout their career. In doing this they abide by the codes provided by their relevant professional regulatory body (Health Professions Council, 2003; General Medical Council, 2006; General Social Care Council, 2002; Nursing and Midwifery Council, 2004). The self-regulation process normally involves a process of periodic review and re-registration to ensure that practitioners continue to meet professional standards with their claim to ongoing development supported by a portfolio of relevant evidence. This information is subject to a process of auditing or gathering of information about practitioners to ensure that regulatory standards are being upheld.

It is important to know and understand your professional requirements for professional self-regulation. To do this you must have read and be familiar with your professional code of conduct and the requirements for CPD published by your relevant professional regulatory body.

Current proposals for change in professional regulation within the NHS (Department of Health, 2006a, b) recommend that the revalidation of professional practice should, in future, be directly linked to the annual appraisal of personal, career and service development as identified in the NHS Knowledge and Skills Framework (Department of Health, 2004). These new proposals create strong links between formative developmental appraisal, the subsequent direction of individual CPD and summative assessment of competence for professional re-registration, with portfolios likely to play a vital role in providing the necessary evidence.

The impact of portfolio development on the learner

Although there are a variety of portfolio models in operation (Smith and Tillema, 2003), McMullan *et al* (2003: 288) give a useful general definition of the portfolio as:

> *a collection of evidence, usually in written form, of both the products and processes of learning. It attests to achievement and personal and professional development by providing critical analysis of its contents.*

This definition is useful because it identifies the main features of portfolios and indicates that a portfolio will normally contain a collection of 'evidence', that demonstrates:

- Any learning achieved and resulting change or proposed change in performance (product). This would, for example, therefore include evidence that demonstrates practice improvement (for example, observation feedback from an assessor, peer review, testimonies) to meet an identified competency, outcome or standard.
- The developmental theoretical and experiential processes (sometimes referred to as the journey) that were undertaken in order to achieve the learning. This might include evidence such as self-assessment of learning needs, action plans, reflective journals, learning logs, reflective writing, self and peer evaluation.
- A critical analysis or narrative of the evidence that explains (normally to assessors) how and where evidence within the portfolio demonstrates achievement. This element may be written within the portfolio or it may be verbally achieved, for example, through a portfolio presentation or a viva voce examination.

Using the above as a guide list what do you think the expectations are of you as a learner when you are completing a portfolio for learning and assessment?

It is important to remember that one of the roles of portfolios in educational programmes is to help facilitate the development of learning skills which enable self-monitoring, self-directed practitioners. Therefore when looking at the list of expectations below there may be aspects that learners new to portfolios may not yet be familiar with and do not know how to achieve. Indeed, as Neades (2003) illustrates, common obstacles to portfolio development include

- lack of experience in portfolio development,
- difficulties in prioritising and organising workload (planning problems),
- difficulties in being disciplined and being self-directed,
- finding it hard to critically appraise practice and own development,
- difficulty collecting evidence so that not enough is available at the summative assessment point,
- coping with the pressure of time – portfolios require time to complete properly.

To avoid these obstacles, it may be useful to use the following list of expectations to make a self-assessment while preparing to start portfolio development. In identifying the aspects that require more learning and support, tutorials can be focused more effectively in meeting individual support needs.

The list below shows some of the expectations or assumptions that might be made of learners when being asked to complete a portfolio for learning and assessment. Did you have some of these in your own list?

Expectations

- Learners have adult learning characteristics (Knowles, 1975) and are self-regulated (Zimmerman, 1989 cited by Dann, 2002). They
  - direct and take responsibility for own learning (self-directed)
  - are self-motivated to achieve
  - are ready to learn – use problems to focus learning
  - use experiences as a source of learning
  - select appropriate learning strategies and opportunities
  - contribute to a positive learning environment
  - are able to choose the type and amount of teaching support needed.
- Learners see learning as an individual process. They
  - recognise that the contents of the portfolio will be individually constructed and therefore different to others
  - use the learning strategies that normally help them learn most effectively according to their learning style
  - choose models and tools which suit them best in their portfolio.
- Learners view learning and assessment as an incremental, developmental process that directs learning. They
  - understand that portfolio activities start at the beginning of the learning experience
  - engage in self-assessment
  - are able to use existing experience and evidence to identify strengths and gaps in own performance
  - can identify support needs and resources for learning
  - are able to identify related learning needs and plan learning aimed at improving weaknesses or gaps in performance
  - actively seek regular opportunities to review own learning and performance and gain feedback from others, eg. mentors, managers, peers and clients.
- Learners are able to reflect in and on practice. They
  - are familiar with using reflective tools for ongoing reflection on experience, eg. journals, diaries and learning logs
  - use dialogue with others to aid the reflective process, e.g. clinical supervision, mentoring
  - understand different 'levels' of reflection and the 'level' expected in the portfolio
  - are familiar with reflective models and writing. Learners are able to analyse critically the contents of a portfolio
  - can provide a written or verbal analysis
  - can explain which pieces of evidence demonstrate the identified outcomes/competency

- can provide a map or cross-reference of this evidence to the different outcomes/competencies.
- Learners are able to prioritise and organise time effectively. They
  - start the portfolios activities as soon as possible to guide appropriate learning
  - ensure that goals and action plans are achievable and realistic through discussion with mentors and lecturers
  - compile the evidence in their portfolios as they collect it and do not leave it all to the end
  - seek support for any areas of uncertainty as early as possible
  - organise any appointments for observations, assessments, feedback and tutorials with lecturers, mentors and supervisors as early as possible
  - get early feedback on reflective writing and critical analysis.

Although these learner expectations may be similar for many portfolios, it is important to note that the model and design of portfolios varies depending on their main purpose (Smith and Tillema, 2003; Endacott *et al*, 2004). This may mean that even if you have completed a portfolio before, you feel new to what is expected of you when you start a new course. In addition, if the academic level of the course is higher than that previously experienced and the portfolio is to be assessed academically, expectations about factors such as the level of critical thinking, analysis and evaluation may be different. Therefore, as well as any competencies that you need to achieve, it is important to understand the academic criteria against which the portfolio is being assessed.

- Find out the assessment criteria for your portfolio. If you are unfamiliar with or unsure about any terms used make sure that you seek clarification from your assessor(s).
- When you have completed a piece of analysis or reflective writing for your portfolio try using the criteria to estimate the feedback that you think you would achieve.
- Gain some assessor feedback and see how this compares with your own.
- Keep referring to any assessment guidelines and criteria throughout the portfolio construction.

Developing study skills and being self-directed

It has been argued that one of the main purposes of a portfolio is to develop in the learner an ability to be a self-directed and lifelong learner and the development of study skills is a vital part of this process. When completing self-assessment, you may have found aspects such as managing time a personal challenge, whereas others may be concerned about writing at an appropriate academic level. You may find it useful to follow the study skills guidance given in *Table 1.1* in order to help you develop these areas. You may also find that your own educational organisation publishes study skills guides and has dedicated study skills support – your tutor can give you more guidance as to the specific facilities available to you. Dedicated study skills support texts will also be available from local libraries.

Snelgrove and Slater (2003) argue that a student's approach to learning is affected by motivations to learn. These can be influenced by the design of the course and the assessments that students have to undertake. For example, learning and assessment which relies more on memorising (rote-learning) rather than understanding has been defined as a surface approach to learning. This type of learning may be motivated by assessments in which information is expected to be reproduced rather than analysed or evaluated and the learning tends to be superficial as a result. On a personal level, high anxiety and lack of interest in the subject have also been identified as causing this type of approach to learning (Cowman, 1998). In contrast, a deep approach to learning is one in which learners seek to understand the meaning of their reading and study, through questioning, challenging and justifying arguments and evidence in relation to previous knowledge and experience (Cowman, 1998).

Because this deep approach to learning is facilitated by experience-based and reflective approaches it is consequently encouraged by portfolio development and assessment. In addition, the research of Mansouri *et al* (2006) highlights the importance of combining a deep and strategic approach to learning (the latter includes the above systematic organisation of study and study time) in achieving a higher level of learning and academic success.

You may find it useful to read Mansouri *et al*'s (2006) article on nursing and midwifery students' approaches to study and learning. The article includes an illustration of items from an inventory indicating individual factors pertaining to deep, surface and strategic approaches to learning.

As well as the approach to learning, individuals are thought to have different preferences for learning or learning styles. Honey and Mumford (1982) developed a typology of experiential learning styles and identified four main types which may be a useful model to explore:

* *Activist*: prefers doing and experiencing
* *Reflector*: prefers to observe and reflect
* *Theorist*: prefers to understand the underlying reasons, concepts and relationships
* *Pragmatist*: prefers active experimentation – having a go to see if something will work

---

Table 1.1. Managing time effectively (Nursing Standard 2002, Bennett 2003)

- *Get to know your library and student support system*
  Make sure that you know and can use your library system effectively as this will reduce time searching for study material. This will include both visiting the library and also understanding the electronic library services that are available to you. Be familiar with the study support available within your learning organisation. This may include support with developing IT skills

- *Develop your IT skills*
  Although you may have a variety of artefacts in your portfolio, there may be an expectation that aspects such as critical reflection and analysis are typed and it will save time if you are able to type these straight onto a computer. In addition, computers can also be useful for filing and storing data such as notes and references for easy recall

- *Prepare a study plan*
  Include details of formal (taught) study periods, work and/or placement periods, independent learning (study) periods and social time. Identify an aim or task for each period of study and study in short (30 minutes maximum) concentrated periods, followed by a short break. Consider whether there are any other times in the day that could be utilised, for example waiting for children or time spent on trains or buses. Include family or other key people in developing your study timetable to ensure that study time has been negotiated with influential others

- *Study in a group*
  Sharing resources and learning with peers in a study group can help you to become more critical in your reading and arguments. Sharing resources also reduces the amount of time that you will need to spend individually searching for information. This can be done electronically, for example, through group e-mail as well as on campus

- *Use tutorial support*
  Anxiety is a major barrier to learning and could prevent you from managing your time effectively, by putting off portfolio learning and activities. This in turn could be detrimental to the successful assessment of the portfolio. If you are anxious about your portfolio assessment it is important to manage that anxiety by seeking tutorial help and support as soon as possible (Price, 2002). Try to keep a focus for your tutorial. Write your questions beforehand and take notes during the tutorial to refer to later

---

Honey and Mumford (1982) suggest that in recognising the area with which we are best aligned we can work to develop the other less developed areas to increase learning effectiveness. While it may be interesting to consider the ways in which you prefer to learn as this may help guide your selection of learning methods and strategies, it is worth noting that there is some criticism of the validity of investigating learning styles, particularly the lack of empirical evidence of their effectiveness (Coffield *et al*, 2004).

Recognising previous learning

Jarvis (2004) states that experiential learning occurs when there is a gap (disjuncture) between learners' previous biographical experiences and the experiences with which they are faced in a new area or aspect of practice. However, in thinking about the new practice, learners should reflect upon and recall previous learning and experience to see whether the knowledge, skills, attitudes, and values previously gained can be transferred into this new situation (Jarvis, 2004). This recognition of previous learning is a very important part of portfolio construction, helping to give learners a greater sense of control and ability to see the development needed from the beginning of their programme (Buchanan, 2004 cited by Roberts, 2006). Feedback from others enhances this self-assessment and critical assessment process (Fitzpatrick, 2006).

However, it is important to recognise that many learners in a completely new learning experience feel that they cannot assess themselves to begin with as they 'do not know what they do not know' and, even though they are prepared to take responsibility for their learning, they will need specific direction and supervision from a supervisor/assessor in order to progress.

Assessment, including self-assessment is discussed in more detail in *Chapter 2*. When you do not know what you need to know, the following strategies can be adopted.

- Make sure you read and understand all the competencies and assessment criteria related to the stage of your course. Discuss these with your instructor and if anything is unclear to you, clarify immediately with your supervisor/assessor.
- Self-assessment:Think about what you have done before; do you have any baseline knowledge or previous experience that you could already apply to these new competencies? Do you have any evidence of previous learning that you could put into your portfolio to support this initial self-assessment?
- Discuss this self-assessment with your supervisor/assessor and gain feedback on it. Your supervisor/assessor may help you to see how some of the skills that you already have act as a baseline or transfer in to these new competencies.

- After your self-assessment, work with your supervisor/assessor to identify specific learning objectives.
- Write an action plan that outlines the actions that you will take in order to achieve the outcome and how you and your assessor will measure achievement. A learning contract may be useful for agreeing any actions that you need to achieve in partnership with others such as mentors, lecturers and peers.
- As you develop greater understanding of the competencies you need to develop you will be able to be more self-directed in recognising the value of previous learning as well as being able to see the gaps between current knowledge and desired competence.

Directing learning

Because portfolio learning is underpinned by adult learning theory, learners are expected to take responsibility for directing their learning according to the specific needs that they have. Indeed it has been suggested that the level of choice and autonomy that this brings may be valued by some learners as a motivator for learning (Pedley and Arber, 1997). Beard (2006) argues that the creation and management of experience is central to the learning process and includes both the need to proactively plan learning and the ability to reflect upon and respond to the unplanned or anticipated experiences through which learning may occur. In managing experience, Beard (2006) suggests that the use of learning plans can be helpful in developing a proactive approach to the creation and management of relevant learning activities and strategies in order to make the most opportunity for learning from an experience. However, it has also been argued that some learners are unused to taking such an active participatory role in their learning and require more facilitation and support from others in order to help direct their learning (Ghazi and Henshaw, 1998). Facilitators therefore will need to support some learners in developing a written action plan that provides a framework to structure their experiential learning.

Action plans are also important tools in the portfolio assessment process because they help the learner to identify and record the ways in which successful achievement will be measured and indicate the type of evidence required for submission in the portfolio. Therefore, within any assessment process, even if learners take full responsibility for developing their action plans, these normally need to be discussed, agreed and countersigned with the assessor. A good action plan should include (Learning and Teaching Scotland, 2006):

- details of intended learning goals and outcomes,
- the actions needed by the learner in order to learn,

- the resources needed to facilitate these actions (for example, this might include other people, time, access),
- the ways in which achievement/success will be measured and by whom.

The first stage of action planning lies with an initial self-assessment. If your portfolio is to be used as an assessment tool, it will help to read and understand the competencies and assessment criteria that are related to the stage of your course and if unclear, these should be discussed with your supervisor/assessor. It is then helpful to consider your existing strengths and weaknesses in relation to these – what you do well, what you have done before, do you have any baseline knowledge or previous experience that you could already apply to these new competencies, do you have any evidence of previous learning that you could put into your portfolio to support this initial self-assessment?

Having established your baseline knowledge and experience, it is now helpful to consider the areas for development, the areas that you need to learn. The next stage of action planning is therefore learning to identify and set the goals that will help to direct this learning. This setting of goals is argued to give learners a greater sense of control over their learning so increasing the internal motivation to learn (Rolheiser *et al*, 2000), and will be discussed in more detail in *Chapter 2*.

Once goals have been identified it is important to identify and record the actions necessary to achieve those goals. These may include both experiential and theoretical learning activities related to the goal. For example, you recognise that in order to achieve your goal you need to observe an aspect of practice, attend a related classroom session and undertake some independent study in order to demonstrate that you have the knowledge necessary to move onto supervised participation in the activity.

It is also important to find a way of recording these planned learning activities as well as any unplanned experiences that occur, and writing a learning log has been identified as a useful activity for this (Barclay, 1996). Brockbank and McGill (1998) refer to a learning log as a privately compiled continuous record of experience throughout a learning programme (and so includes records and thoughts on learning gained from both theoretical and experiential elements). They stress that a learning log is frequently highly personal, private and confidential, with learners controlling which elements they are willing to share with others. A learning log, while recording the learning process and linking it to learning goals, may therefore be more likely to appear as chosen excerpts in a portfolio rather than presented in its entirety (Brockbank and McGill, 1998).

Becoming reflective

Critical reflection on practice is an important aspect of the experiential learning process, helping all practitioners to develop their knowledge to improve their own performance (Rolfe *et al*, 2001). Within the portfolio there will need to be evidence that the learner has developed a reflective approach to practice. This could include evidence of verbal reflection through peer review and supervision sessions or examples of reflective writing such as diaries or writing around critical incidents that have become an emergent learning experience. The assumptions of writing in order to learn, suggest that as an activity it aids understanding, thinking and learning. Models of reflection can be utilised to help learners start to structure their writing enabling them to think not only about the description of the event, but also analysing and evaluating it so that learning can be identified (Rolfe *et al*, 2001). Examples of reflective models can be found in *Chapter 3*.

Summary

This chapter has outlined some of the context underlying the changing nature of professional education and its implications for portfolio development. The importance for professionals to have self-regulatory abilities and to be lifelong learners in order to maintain competent practice at a time of rapid global change has been identified. Portfolios have been identified as a tool that can both facilitate and direct a lifelong learning approach because they are centred on directing and recording individual learning and development over time. In order to make the most of portfolio learning and assessment it is important for students to develop their ability to be independent and self-directed reflective learners, able to direct their learning through appropriate action planning.

References

Barclay J (1996) Assessing the benefits of learning logs. *Education and Training* **38**(2): 30–8

Baume D, Yorke M, Coffey M (2004) What is happening when we assess, and how can we use our understanding of this to improve assessment? *Assessment and Evaluation in Higher Education* **29**(4): 451–77

Beard C (2006) *Experiential Learning: A Handbook of Best Practice for Educators and Trainers*. Kogan Page, London

Bennett C (2003) On course for success *Nursing Standard* **18**(7): 32

Brockbank A, McGill I (1998) *Facilitating Reflective Learning in Higher Education*. SRHE and Open University, Buckingham

Buchanan EA (2004) Online assessment in higher education: Strategies to systematically evaluate student learning. In Howard C, Schenk K, Discenza R (eds) *Distance Learning and University Effectiveness: Changing Educational Paradigms for Online Learning*. Information Science Publishing

Cadman C, Brewer J (2001) Emotional intelligence: A vital prerequisite for recruitment in nursing. *J Nursing Manag* **9**(6): 321–4

Clarke CL, Wilcockson J (2001) Professional and organizational learning: Analysing the relationship with the development of practice. *J Adv Nursing* 34(2): 264–72

Coffield F, Moseley D, Hall E, Ecclestone K (2004) *Learning Styles and Pedagogy in Post-16 Learning. A Systematic and Critical Review.* Learning and Skills Research Centre, London

Corcoran J, Nicholson C (2004) Learning portfolios – evidence of learning: An examination of students' perspectives. *British Association of Critical Care Nurses, Nursing in Critical Care* **9**(5): 230–7

Cowman S (1998) The approaches to learning of student nurses in the Republic of Ireland and Northern Ireland. *J Adv Nursing* **28**(4): 899–910

Crick,R.D and Wilson, K (2005) Being a learner: A virtue for the 21st Century. *Brit J Educational Studies* **53**(3): 359–74

Dall 'Alba G (2004) Understanding professional practice: Investigations before and after an educational programme. *Studies in Higher Education* **29**: 679–92

Dann R (2002) *Promoting Assessment as Learning: Improving the Learning Process.* Routledge Falmer, London

Davis C (2000) *Interpreting Professional Self-Regulation: A History of the United Kingdom Central Council for Nursing.* Routledge, Florence, KY

Dewar B, Walker E (1999) Experiential learning: Issues for supervision. *J Adv Nursing* **30**(6): 1459–67

Department for Education and Skills (2003) *The Future of Higher Education.* Department for Education and Skills, London

Department of Health (1999) *Making a Difference: Strengthening the Nursing, Midwifery and Health Visiting Contribution to Health and Healthcare.* Department of Health, London

Department of Health (2000) *The NHS Plan: A Plan for Investment, a Plan for Reform.* Department of Health, London

Department of Health (2001) *Working Together, Learning Together.* Department of Health, London

Department of Health (2004) *The NHS Knowledge and Skills Framework (NHS KSF) and the Development Review Process.* Department of Health, London

Department of Health (2006a) *The Regulation of the Non-medical Healthcare Professions.* Department of Health, London

Department of Health (2006b) *Good doctors, Safer Patients: Proposals to Strengthen the System to Assure and Improve the Performance of Doctors and to Protect the Safety of Patients.* Department of Health, London

Edwards R (1997) *Changing Places? Flexibility, Lifelong Learning and a Learning Society.* Routledge, London

Endacott R, Gray MA, Jasper MA, McMullan M, Miller C, Scholes J, Webb C (2004) Using portfolios in the assessment of learning and competence: The impact of four models. *Nurse Education in Practice* **4**: 250–7

Eraut M (1992) Developing the knowledge base: A process perspective on professional education. In Barnett R (ed) *Learning to Effect*. Buckingham, Society for Research into Higher Education (SRHE) and Open University Press cited by Taylor I (1997) Developing Learning in Professional Education. Partnerships for Practice. SRHE and Open University Press

Fitzpatrick J (2006) Self-assessment as a strategy to provoke integrative learning within a professional degree programme. *Learning in Health and Social Care* **5**(1): 23–34

Freshwater D, Stickley T (2004) The heart of the art: Emotional intelligence in nurse education. *Nursing Inquiry* **11**(2): 91–8

Frowe I (2005) Professional Trust. *Brit J Educational Studies* **53**(1): 34–53

General Medical Council (2006) *Good Medical Practice*. From http://www.gmc-uk.org/guidance/good_medical_practice/index.asp Accessed 2/01/07

General Social Care Council (2002) *Codes of Practice for Social Care Workers and Employers*. General Social Care Council, London

Ghaye T, Ghaye K (1998) *Teaching and Learning Through Critical Reflective Practice*. David Fulton, London

Ghazi F, Henshaw L (1998) How to keep students motivated. *Nursing Standard* **13**: 43–8

Gonsci A (1994) Competency based assessment in the professions in Australia. *Assessment in Education* **1**: 27–44

Gopee N (2001) Lifelong learning in nursing: Perceptions and realities. *Nurse Education Today* **21**(8): 607–15

Health Professions Council (2003) *Standards of Conduct, Performance and Ethics*. From: http://www.hpc-uk.org/publications/standards/index.asp?id=38

Honey P, Mumford A (1982) *Manual of Learning Styles*. P Honey, London

Jarvis P (2004) *Adult Education and Lifelong Learning. Theory and Practice* (3rd edn) Routledge Falmer, London

Knowles M (1975) *Self-Directed Learning: A Guide for Learners and Teachers*. Follet, Chicago

Learning and Teaching Scotland (2006) *Action plan – Definition*. From: http://www.ltscotland.org.uk/sharedglossary/actionplan.asp. Accessed: 17/01/07

Mansouri P, Soltani F, Rahemi S, Nasab MM, Ayatollahi AR, Nekooeian AA (2006) Nursing and midwifery students' approaches to study and learning. *J Adv Nursing* **54**(3): 351–8

McMullan M, Endacott R, Gray MA, Miller CML, Scholes J, Webb C (2003) Portfolios and assessment of competence: A review of the literature. *J Adv Nursing* **41**(3): 283–94

Moon JA (2004) *A Handbook of Reflective and Experiential Learning, Theory and Practice*. Routledge Falmer, London

National Committee of Inquiry into Higher Education (1997) *Higher Education in the Learning Society* (Dearing report). From: http://www.leeds.ac.uk/educol/ncihe/

Neades BL (2003) Professional portfolios: All you need to know and were afraid to ask. *A & E Nursing* **11**: 49–55

Nursing and Midwifery Council (2004) *The NMC Code of Professional Conduct: Standards for Conduct, Performance and Ethics.* NMC, London

Nursing Standard (2002) Effective learning number 2: Planning effective study. *Nursing Standard* **17**(4): 1–3

Pedley GE, Arber A (1997) Nursing students' response to self-directed learning: An evaluation of a learning process applying Jarvis' framework. *J Adv Nursing* **25**: 405–11

Price, B (2002) Gaining the most from your tutor. *Nursing Standard* **16**(25): 40–4

Roberts TS (2006) *Self, Peer and Group Assessment in E-Learning.* Hershey Information Science Publishing, London

Rolfe G, Freshwater D, Jasper M (2001) *Critical Reflection for Nursing and the Helping Professions.* Palgrave Macmillan, Basingstoke

Rolheiser C, Bowewr B, Stevahn L (2000) *Portfolio Organizer: Succeeding with Portfolios in Your Classroom.* Association for Supervision and Curriculum Development

Schon D (1983) *The Reflective Practitioner.* Basic Books, New York

Smith K, Tillema H (2003) Clarifying different types of portfolio use. *Assessment and Evaluation in Higher Education* **28**(6): 625–48

Snelgrove S, Slater J (2003) Approaches to learning: Psychometric testing of a study process questionnaire. *J Adv Nursing* **43**(5): 496–505

Stuart CC (2003) *Assessment, Supervision and Support in Clinical Practice: A Guide for Nurses and Midwives.* Churchill Livingstone, London

UKCC (1999) *Fitness for Practice. The Report of the UKCC Commission for Nursing and Midwifery Education.* UKCC, London

Watson R, Stimpson Topping A, Porock D (2002) Clinical competence assessment in nursing: A systematic review of the literature. *J Adv Nursing* **39**(5): 421–31

Zimmerman BJ (1989) Models of self-regulated learning and academic achievement. In Zimmerman BJ, Schunk DH (eds) *Self Regulated Learning and Academic Achievement.* Springer Verlag, New York

CHAPTER 2

Assessment

Val Nixon

Introduction

This chapter discusses the use of the portfolio as an assessment strategy within higher education. A brief discussion of experiential learning is offered and examples are given of learning taxonomies that can be used to monitor and assess progress both in knowledge and skills acquisition.

At the start of any learning journey it is important to reflect on current skills, knowledge, experience and understanding to give a starting point on which to build and develop. There is a vast array of self-assessment strategies and structured planning tools that can be used to facilitate this process. It is beyond the scope of this chapter to discuss all these strategies, but commonly used tools such as SWOT (strengths, weaknesses, opportunites and threats) analysis, goal setting and action planning will be discussed alongside examples of how to use these tools effectively to achieve the desired outcomes.

As most of your development and learning may be gained through experiential learning, supervision and mentorship is imperative to guide and support your learning journey. The role and expectations of a mentor/student partnership will be discussed, including the process of setting ground rules for the partnership and the development of learning contracts.

What is assessment?

Assessment is a vital part of the education process (Rowntree, 1977) and, as such, it deserves meticulous attention during the curriculum design process. The process of assessment is highly complex and subjective, and there are many diverse views on assessment leading to general confusion about what assessment is and what it is not. The Higher Education Quality Control (HEQC) (1996) guidelines suggest that assessment is the exercise of judgement on the quality of students' work as a way of supporting student learning and of appraising its outcomes. Nicklin and Kenworthy (1995: 69) provide a relatively simple yet unambiguous definition of assessment as:

> *A measurement that directly relates to the quality and quantity of learning and as such is concerned with student progress and attainment.*

Regardless of the many definitions, Quinn (2000) identifies three basic aims of assessment:

- It should assess student performance in relation to the aims of the particular programme in question.
- It should be regarded as an integral component of the teaching and learning process, and not simply as a means of measuring attainment.
- It should encourage students to undertake self-assessment and reflection on their learning.

The aims of assessment as identified by Quinn (2000) appear to fulfil the requirements for using portfolios as an assessment strategy within higher education as they capture important elements that are aimed towards facilitating a student-led approach.

The portfolio as an assessment strategy

There are a variety of strategies within higher education that address the aims of assessment, and nurse educators need objective relevant tools for measuring the quality and quantity of student learning, progress and achievement. One method of achieving this is through educational portfolios. One of the most quoted definitions of portfolios is by Brown (1992: 1) who states that a portfolio is

a private collection of evidence which demonstrates the continuing acquisition of skills, knowledge, understanding and achievement. It is both retrospective and prospective, as well as reflecting the current stage of development and activity of the individual.

This suggests that a portfolio can contain material from a variety of sources, chosen by the individual, which is capable of conveying to others the qualities, competencies and abilities of the owner, as well as providing an indication of potential development (Brown, 1992).

The term portfolio is used within the professional and higher educational arenas, but there has been some confusion as to whether or not the term means the same thing in each. Professionally, in order to fulfil post-registration education and practice requirements (PREP), it is mandatory for all qualified nurses, midwives and community public health nurses to maintain a personal professional profile (PPP) (Nursing and Midwifery Council, 2006a). As a professional tool the portfolio will enable you to record your career and post-registration education and practice (Nursing and Midwifery Council, 2006a). The documentary evidence with an explanatory commentary may be used to assist you in reflecting on your own professional practice as well as demonstrating to others the quality of the work you have been doing. It provides a clear and concise framework within which a comprehensive resource can be built up that will be useful when:

- applying for a new post,
- compiling a curriculum vitae,
- seeking accreditation for prior learning and experience,
- participating in performance review,
- building a personal development profile,
- meeting the statutory requirements for renewing Nursing and Midwifery Council registration.

Within higher education, portfolios are seen as a valuable learning strategy in educational programmes. They are used to describe multidimensional methods of presenting information, usually about the students' achievements, attributes or performances (Frith and Macintosh, 1984). There is a variety of information that can be used as evidence within a portfolio and this is discussed in *Chapter 3*. As an assessment strategy, Baume (2001: 9) defines a portfolio as a

> *structured collection comprising labelled evidence and critical reflection on that evidence...It is presented to show evidence of that learning. It may additionally comprise an explicit claim or demonstration that specified outcomes have been achieved.*

A portfolio therefore enables an assessor to measure student learning, acts as a tool for reflective thinking, illustrates critical analytical skills and evidence of self-directed learning and provides a collection of detailed evidence of a person's competence. Furthermore, the portfolio approach differs from the traditional approach of passive, teacher-led learning as it is more focused towards a student-led approach with the emphasis on experiential learning, where the student is actively involved with the reality of what is being studied (Kolb, 1984; Quinn, 1998; Redfern, 1998).

Experiential learning and experiential taxonomies

I hear, I know
I see, I remember
I do, I understand   Confucius (551BC–479BC)

Experiential learning can be traced back to the 1930s to educational philosopher John Dewey (1938) who believed that all genuine education comes through experience. Within the past 20 years experiential learning has become firmly established in nursing, midwifery and community public health curricula. As a result, it has become a contemporary approach to nurse education as facilitation of learning in the clinical environment is mainly learning from experience (Downie and Basford, 1997).

A simplistic view of experiential learning is that it is learning that results from experience, essentially learning by doing, rather that listening to other people or reading (Quinn, 2000). Taking this simplistic view, assessment of learning in clinical practice will therefore be undertaken through experiential taxonomies. Several taxonomies have been devised that classify learning objectives including the cognitive taxonomy (Bloom, 1956), the affective taxonomy (Bloom *et al*, 1964), and the psychomotor taxonomies of Simpson (1966) and Harrow (1972).

These classifications, or taxonomies delineate the consequence of the educative process into three divisions or domains:

- The cognitive domain: use of information and knowledge.
- The affective domain: attitudes, emotions and values.
- The psychomotor domain: doing and motor skills.

These have provided useful tools for curriculum development for both educationalists and students. Yet each of these taxonomies addresses only one aspect of human experience. Although one can look at human experience through the cognitive taxonomy, the affective taxonomy, or a psychomotor taxonomy, none of these addresses the whole of human experience. Steinaker and Bell (1979) developed an experiential taxonomy that incorporates the totality of human experience. They view the total human experience as essential and their ideas were based on a definition in Webster's New World Dictionary of the American Language (1976), which defines experience as 'living through an event or events'. The 'living through' events is viewed as involving the total personality (Steinaker and Bell, 1979). The taxonomy has five basic categories and a number of subcategories. Through these categories a natural and logical progression is possible, leading to the planned outcome, namely learning. The categories are intrinsically linked together and an individual can move through an experience from exposure to dissemination, whether the experience is positive or negative, and through this process from inability to achievement.

Steinaker and Bell's categories of the experiential taxonomy

The following categories are adapted from Steinaker and Bell's experiential taxonomy (1979).

1.0 *Exposure*: Consciousness of an experience. This involves two levels of exposure and a readiness for further experience:
   1.1 Sensory
   1.2 Response
   1.3 Readiness.
2.0 *Participation*: The decision to become physically a part of an experience. There are two levels of interaction within this category:
   2.1 Representation
      2.1.1 Covertly
      2.1.2 Overtly
   2.2 Modification.
3.0 *Identification*: The coming together of the learner and the idea (objective) in an emotional and intellectual context for the achievement of the objective:
   3.1 Reinforcement
   3.2 Emotional
   3.3 Personal
   3.4 Sharing.
4.0 *Internalisation*: The participant moves from identification to internalisation when the experience begins to affect the life-style of the participant. There are two levels in this category:
   4.1 Expansion
   4.2 Intrinsic.
5.0 *Dissemination*: The experience moves beyond internalisation to dissemination. It goes beyond the positive sharing that began at level 3.0 (identification) and involves two levels of activity:
   5.1 Informal
   5.2 Homiletic.
6.0 *Exposure*: Consciousness of an experience. This involves two levels of exposure and a readiness for further experience.

It must be noted that the categories of this taxonomy are stated in positive terms while an experience can bring forth either positive or negative reactions. For the purpose of teaching and learning, a positive statement of categories is essential. *Table 2.1* demonstrates a number of learning behaviours for each category that will enable you to progress naturally through the stages to achieve your planned outcome.

Benner's skills acquisition model

Another model that sees learning through experience is Benner's (1984) skills acquisition model. This model draws on the work of Dreyfus and Dreyfus (1980). The Dreyfus model posits that in the acquisition and development of

Table 2.1. Categories of Steinaker and Bell's experiential taxonomy

Exposure
Student is exposed
to the experience

- Shows an awareness but lacks knowledge and skills
- Listens, observes, asks questions
- Reacts to the experience and recognises limitations and responsibilities
- Reflects on learning experience and explores the implications of these reflections

Participation
Student can
reproduce the activity
encountered at the
exposure level

- Begins to articulate underlying rational skills for the activity
- Shows recall of ideas and concepts
- Introduces and discusses background information
- Practises under supervision in a standardised way
- Uses appropriate interpersonal behaviour

Identification
Student is able to
carry out the activity
competently

- Recognises and explains situations where the activity is applicable
- Able to assess own strengths and limitations
- Utilises theory and research in relation to carrying out the activity
- Beginning to show initiative, recognises standards, values and qualities required

Internalisation
Student identifies
with the activity so
it becomes second
nature

- Shows confidence in own activity
- Able to reflect experience in an objective manner
- Able to apply new knowledge to a new situation
- Shows creativity
- Utilises research in relation to the activity
- Undertakes clinical skills in safe and consistent manner

Dissemination
Student acts as role
model by informing
and promoting
experience to others

- Competent, demonstrates ability to teach others
- Illustrates motivational abilities in relation to others
- Is able to carry out the activity in complex unfamiliar situations
- Acts as a role model
- Is able to discuss the wider influences, social and economic, and how these impact on practice

a skill, a student passes through five levels of proficiency: novice, advanced beginner, competent, proficient and expert and that the different levels reflect changes in the three general aspects of skilled performance. One is a movement from reliance on abstract principles to the use of past concrete experience as paradigms. The second is a change in the learner's perception of the demand situation, in which it is seen less and less as a compilation of equally relevant bits, and more and more as a complete whole in which only certain parts are relevant. The third is a passage from detached observer to involved performer. The performer no longer stands outside the situation but is now engaged in the situation. Drawing from this model Benner (1984) describes the performance characteristics at each level of development and identifies, in general terms, the teaching/learning needs at each level.

Stage 1: Novice: Beginners have had no experience of situations on which to draw and rules and regulations are extremely limited and inflexible. This can apply to both students in training and to experienced nurses who move into an unfamiliar clinical area. It is important at this stage to give learners rules and regulations to guide their performance. This can be achieved through the principles and theory learned in a classroom but context-dependent judgements and skill can be acquired only in real situations (Dreyfus, 1982).

Adherence to principles and rules, however, does not help the nurse to decide what is relevant in a nursing situation, and may thus lead to unsuccessful performance. The novice will require one-to-one expert support to validate understanding of care parameters and patient outcomes (Latham and Fahey, 2006).

Stage 2: Advanced beginner: Unlike principles and rules, aspects are overall characteristics of a situation that can only be identified by experience of that situation. Advanced beginners can demonstrate marginally acceptable performance gained from sufficient prior experience (or pointed out to them by a mentor). For example, when performing the skills of obtaining a patient's vital signs (blood pressure, pulse and temperature) the advanced beginner will discriminate between normal and abnormal recordings but may not be able focus on the more advanced skills of judging the relative importance of different aspects of the situation that may result in abnormal findings. The advanced beginner needs adequate support from supervisors, mentors and colleagues in the practice setting. This will provide a safe environment for questions and increase confidence, enhance communication and validate clinical judgement to help the student to see a broader picture (Latham and Fahey, 2006).

Stage 3: Competent: This stage is characterised by conscious, deliberate planning based upon analysis and careful deliberation of situations. Competent nurses are able to identify priorities and manage their own work. Benner (1984) suggests that the competent professional can benefit at this stage from learning activities that centre on decision-making, planning and co-ordinating patient care. For example, when interviewing patients the competent nurse will obtain subjective data but also consciously observe a patient's physical and psychosocial behaviour. This will help the competent nurse to gain an overall analysis in order to determine priorities to plan and manage care that is effective and responsive to the patient's needs. Educationally, experiential learning opportunities will encourage further development (Latham and Fahey, 2006).

Stage 4: Proficient: Characteristically, the proficient nurse is able to perceive situations holistically and at this stage the key word is perception. The perspective is not thought out but 'presents itself' based upon experience and recent events (Benner, 1984). The proficient nurse learns from experience what typical events to expect in a given situation and how plans need to be modified in response to these events. Because of this experience-based ability to recognise the whole situation, the proficient nurse can now recognise when the expected normal picture does not materialise. Holistic understanding improves the nurse's decision making and it becomes less laboured. Unlike the competent nurse, the proficient nurse will be able to consider fewer options and focus directly on the most relevant aspects of a problem. Proficient performance is normally found in nurses who have worked within a specific area of nursing for several years. Inductive teaching strategies, such as case studies, are most useful for nurses at this stage (Quinn, 2000).

Stage 5: Expert: Expert performers no longer rely on an analytical principle to connect their understanding of the situation to an appropriate action. The expert nurse with an enormous background of experience, should have an intuitive grasp of each situation and zero in on the direct problem without wasteful considerations of a large range of unnecessary, alternative diagnoses and solutions. Expert, intuitive nurses cannot always give a rationale for their actions and capturing descriptions of expert performance is difficult because this stage is characterised by a deep understanding and intuitive grasp of the total situation. However, it must be noted that this is not to say that the expert never uses analytical tools. Highly skilled analytical ability is necessary for those situations with which the nurse has had no previous experience. In addition, analytical tools are also necessary for those times when the expert gets a wrong grasp of the situation and finds that events and behaviour are not occurring as expected. Expert clinicians are not difficult to recognise because they frequently make clinical judgements or manage complex clinical situations in a truly remarkable way. Benner (1984) suggests that a crucial incident technique is a useful way of attempting to evaluate expert practice, but considers that not all nurses are capable of becoming experts.

The above are two commonly used experiential taxonomies. There are many more that have not been discussed in this book which you may wish to explore. However, the chosen taxonomy that is used within a module or course should be applicable to the learning outcomes and achievable.

Learning outcomes

As an assessment strategy, the evidence within an educational portfolio that demonstrates that learning has occurred must be directly related to learning outcomes. Learning outcomes and assessment strategies are two sets of statements that should be linked together so that assessment strategies are appropriate to facilitate the achievement of the learning outcomes. For example, the more general the learning outcome statement is, the more detailed will the assessment criteria need to be to support achievement of this learning outcome. The principal purpose of learning outcomes concerns standards of student learning, and the relationship of learning to assessment. They are derived from the educational aims of a programme, but are stated in terms of the capabilities that students should attain as a result of instruction (Quinn, 2000). In terms of a definition, according to Moon (2000: 56) a learning outcome is:

> *A statement of what a learner is expected to know, understand and be able to do at the end of a period of learning and of how that learning is to be demonstrated. Learning outcomes are linked to the relevant level and since they should generally be assessable they should be written in terms of how the learning should be represented.*

This definition clearly states that the learning outcomes must reflect a level of learning. Lower levels such as levels 1 and 2 are depicted by the ability to define and describe, whereas higher levels (levels 3 and 4) are those that demonstrate an advanced level of mastery in relation to deductive reasoning skills, critical analysis, synthesis and creative thoughts (Brown, 1992). In addition, they should be relevant to that level and therefore it is not appropriate to use the same learning outcomes for a module that may be delivered at two different levels. It is acceptable for the teaching of a module to be common to students at two levels, and even the actual assessment task can be similar, but the learning outcomes and the assessment criteria will reflect the actual level and will differ between two modules. Examples of learning outcomes for levels 2 and 3 are shown in *Table 2.2*.

Self-assessment against learning outcomes

When commencing a new programme of study, the learning outcomes may appear daunting because more often than not, they are written at a level of abstraction to accommodate a wide range of clinical situations (Scholes *et al*, 2004). This may appear confusing because of the terminology that is used to explain what you have to achieve. In addition, you may question how you are going to achieve the learning outcomes. This may be due to a

---

Table 2.2. Example of learning outcomes – Levels 2 and 3

Learning outcome: Level 2
- Describe and demonstrate knowledge of anatomy and physiology and apply the principles of pathophysiology of the respiratory system
- Demonstrate the ability to assess, plan and deliver care that is responsive, flexible, relevant and effective in relation to a patient with a respiratory ailment
- Discuss the appropriate evidence-based strategies in the application of treatment to a patient with a respiratory ailment using departmental and national guidelines and protocols

Learning outcome: Level 3
- Demonstrate a detailed knowledge of anatomy and physiology and apply the principles of pathophysiology of the respiratory system
- Demonstrate the ability to assess, analyse and synthesise data to plan and deliver care that is responsive, flexible, relevant and effective in relation to a patient with a respiratory ailment
- Evaluate critically and apply appropriate evidence-based strategies in the application of treatment to a patient with a respiratory ailment using departmental and national guidelines and protocols

---

variety of personal or professional issues such as limited time for study or limited knowledge and skills in relation to the subject matter. On the other hand, you may have a deeper understanding or a wider knowledge base of the subject outcomes and therefore positively identify how you will achieve them. Whatever your feelings, ideas, knowledge, skills, clinical experience, strengths and weaknesses are at the time, capturing these can be extremely valuable. This is the start of the process of self-assessment and will inevitably be the beginning of your learning journey.

Educational portfolios, as an assessment strategy, promote the use of self-assessment. According to Boud (1995) self-assessment occurs when learners make judgements about aspects of their own performance and it is an important skill for lifelong learning. Through monitoring your performance and reflecting on your identified learning needs you should be able to identify what is known, what remains to be known and what is needed to bridge the gap between the two. In addition it promotes motivation to learn as you will have a greater ownership and investment of the learning you are undertaking (Brown and Knight, 1994). Assessment does not then become a process that is undertaken by educational and/or clinical assessors, but it is a participative process in which you, as a student, become involved. Boud (1990) supports this view as he argues that self-assessment is fundamental to all aspects of learning in the belief that learning is an active endeavour and thus it is only the learner who can learn and implement decisions about his or her own learning: all other forms of assessment are therefore subordinate to it.

Methods and tools of self-assessment can be varied within a portfolio. Boud (1992) describes a self-assessment regime in which the student should:

- set goals,
- specify the criteria that define whether those goals have been met,
- describe the evidence to be presented claiming goals have been met,
- set out a case for claiming that the goals have been met,
- action plan to follow from their evaluation.

Before starting a self-assessment regime it is advisable first to complete a SWOT analysis.

SWOT analysis

SWOT stands for strengths, weaknesses, opportunities and threats. A SWOT analysis is a critical self-analysis and summarises where you are right now. It acts as a basis for future growth and includes internal factors (strengths and weaknesses) and external factors (opportunities and threats) that may develop or inhibit learning. When completing a SWOT analysis you should be able to list several strengths in terms of your study habits, knowledge, skills, clinical experience and also strengths of your personality more generally. For example, being a sociable person may not relate directly to your studies, but it is a valuable strength which will help you to be successful as a student and later as an employee. On the other hand, you may be a very reflective person – a deep thinker. This is a very different strength, but no less of an advantage to you. It is important to be positive about these strengths, so if in doubt, add them to your list.

Under weaknesses, you should list any areas of your knowledge, skills, experience, personality or behaviour that you would like to strengthen. If you are a sociable person, this might be the need to develop the habit of private study – hard for someone who likes to talk and listen.

At the start of your journey you will have some clear ideas about your strengths and perhaps some of your weaker areas/limitations too. It is now time to pull these together and list them in your SWOT analysis. Once you have listed key issues you should have a clear idea of where you are starting from and how to work towards achieving the learning outcomes. This will enable you to identify the opportunities and threats (external factors) that would smooth the progress of, or impede, development. It is important to note that identification

Table 2.3. Example of a SWOT analysis

Strengths
- Basic knowledge of anatomy and physiology of the respiratory system
- Basic understanding of pathophysiology
- Previous clinical placement on a respiratory ward
- Knowledge of learning outcomes to be achieved
- Understanding the importance and interpretation of vital signs (temperature, pulse, respiratory rate, blood pressure and oxygen saturation)
- Basic general awareness of evidence-based practice
- Awareness of national guidelines, eg. NICE, SIGN, etc.
- Good communicator
- Motivated to learn new experiences and knowledge
- Ability to work individually
- Good team worker
- Able to recognise when support and guidance is needed

Weaknesses
- Limited theoretical knowledge of a wide range of respiratory diseases
- Minimal clinical experience of assessing and managing patients with respiratory problems
- No knowledge of breath sounds
- Limited awareness of evidence-based practice in relation to treatment for various respiratory diseases
- Limited critical thinking skills particularly when evaluating evidence-based strategies for treatment
- Poor time management skills
- Easily distracted
- Poor concentration

Opportunities
- Clinical placement on a respiratory ward
- Regular contact with the experts in placement area
- To visit other respiratory departments
- To observe and participate with listening to breath sounds under the supervision of a chest physiotherapist
- To work with mentor and observe and participate with assessment and management of patients with a variety of respiratory problems
- To observe clinical nurse specialist in respiratory nursing
- Supernumery status
- Protected study time
- To discuss and reflect on clinical experience and knowledge with mentor

Threats
- Busy environment on the ward
- Limited supervision from mentor – being thrown in at the deep end
- Working with different members of the team on a regular basis
- Not given supernumery status and included as a team member
- Pressures of looking after a family
- Limited theoretical knowledge and clinical experience may demotivate learning
- A wide subject area to learn in the allocated time
- Not suited to respiratory medicine/ nursing

of weaknesses and threats should not be viewed negatively but rather used to identify strengths and opportunities to overcome your weaknesses and threats. For example, *Table 2.3* illustrates a SWOT analysis that is directly linked to the learning outcomes in *Table 2.2*. In the weaknesses section, limited knowledge of a wide range of respiratory diseases has been identified. The identified strength to overcome this weakness is a basic understanding of anatomy, physiology and pathophysiology as this is a starting point on which to advance your knowledge. A threat identified that may hinder learning is pressures of looking after a family. However, protected study time and supernumery status in the clinical environment will be viewed as a positive opportunity to overcome this by making effective use of time.

Goal setting

Goal setting involves establishing a standard or objective to serve as the aim of your actions (Schunk, 2001). Bandura (1997) suggests that goals enhance self-regulation through their effects on motivation, learning, self-efficacy (perceived capabilities for learning or performing actions at given levels), and self-evaluations of progress. Goals are involved across the different phases of self-regulation: planning (setting a goal and deciding on goal strategies); performance control (employing goal-directed actions and monitoring performance); and self-reflection (evaluating one's goal progress and adjusting strategies to ensure success) (Zimmerman, 1998). Goals also direct your attention to relevant task features, behaviours to be performed, and outcomes to be achieved. In addition they should guide you to become more focused, to select and apply appropriate strategies and to monitor your goal progress by comparing your current knowledge, skills and performance with the goal. Initially you must make a commitment to attain a goal because performance will not be affected without this commitment (Locke and Latham, 1990).

The way in which you develop goals strongly affects their effectiveness. When setting goals that are mapped against the learning outcomes it is important to set performance goals as opposed to outcome goals. Performance goals reflect your performance, knowledge and skills towards achieving learning outcomes whereas outcome goals are more general and reflect the end result. For example, to assess competently a patient who presents with a respiratory problem would be viewed as an outcome goal and hence, vulnerable to failure. This would be because factors beyond your control, such as busy ward environment, limited supervision, personal reasons, etc., may prevent this achievement and there is nothing more dispiriting as failing to achieve goals for reasons beyond your control. In contrast, performance goals, put simply, enable you to move from outcome goals to more specific, achievable goals which will be based on personal performance, skills or knowledge to be acquired. These tend to be more attainable as control can be maintained over your achievement, which consequently leads to satisfaction and self-confidence (see *Figure 2.1*).

To strengthen general outcome goals into powerful and effective performance goals the use of the SMART (specific, measurable, achievable, relevant/realistic, timely) mnemonic is important.

Specific goals

Specific goals are the what, why, and how of the SMART model:

- What are you going to do? Use action words such as direct, organise, co-ordinate, lead, develop, plan, build, etc.
- Why is this important to do at this time?
- What do you want ultimately to accomplish?
- How are you going to do it?

If you set a precise goal, put in dates, times and amounts so that achievement can be measured. In this way you know the exact goal to be achieved, and can take satisfaction from having achieved it. Goals that incorporate specific performance standards are more likely to enhance self-regulation and activate self-evaluations than general goals such as 'do my best' or 'try hard' (Locke and Latham, 1990). Specific goals raise performance because they specify the amount of effort required for success and boost self-efficacy by providing a clear standard against which to determine progress

Measurable goals

Goals can be so vague that they may not be useful or of any real benefit in the learning process, and can make it difficult to ascertain whether such goals have been achieved. If achievement cannot be measured, then your self-confidence will not benefit from goal setting, nor can you observe progress towards a greater goal. Set precise, quantitative goals and if you achieve all conditions of a measurable goal, then you can be confident and comfortable in its achievement. If you consistently fail to meet a measurable goal, then you can adjust it or analyse the reason for failure and take appropriate action to improve skills.

Achievable goals

When you identify goals that are most important to you, you begin to develop

Name of student:		Name of mentor:		Date:	
Outcome goal	Performance goal	Action required	Weaknesses/threats	Strengths/opportunities	Achieved by
To develop and demonstrate a competent level (identification) of assessing a patient with a respiratory problem.	1. To increase my knowledge of anatomy and physiology of respiratory system. 2. To increase my knowledge of pathophsiology of common respiratory problems, eg. chest infection, pneumonia, COPD, asthma. 3. To increase my confidence with assessing patients. 4. To develop effective communication skills to obtain accurate information.	1. To attend library and review literature for a minimum of 4 hr/wk. 2. To observe qualified nurses undertaking assessments – a minimum of 10 observations of 4 common presenting conditions. 3. To listen to patient's current and past medical history – minimum of 4 common conditions. 4. To participate in undertaking a minimum of 10 assessments of patients with respiratory problems with respiratory problems under supervision. 5. To reflect on my current knowledge and skills, and discuss with mentor areas for development.	Time to study. Poor time management skills Time to study wide range of respiratory illnesses. Busy ward environment. Limited understanding of pathophysiology that may hinder my understanding of signs and symptoms. Limited supervision from mentor. Not given supernumery status therefore limited time to observe other healthcare professionals. No time to reflect with mentor .	Protected study time. Basic understanding of anatomy and physiology Clinical placement on respiratory ward. Supernumery status. Working with mentor and other expert healthcare professionals.	1. 14.01.06 2. 14.01.06 3. 21.01.06 4. 02.02.06 5. 10.02.06
	To complete a patient assessment confidently and competently under supervision.	To complete an assessment of a patient admitted with a respiratory condition.	Time. Limited supervision from mentor. Lack of confidence.		28.02.06

Figure 2.1. Example of goal setting and action plan.

ways you can achieve them. You may develop the attitudes, abilities, skills, and financial capacity to reach them. You begin seeing previously overlooked opportunities to bring yourself closer to the achievement of your goals. Any goals you set which are unrealistic, probably will not inspire your commitment to their completion. Although you may start with the best of intentions, the overwhelming feeling that 'it's just too much', means your subconscious will keep reminding you of this fact and may stop you from being motivated to give it your best.

Realistic goals

This is not a synonym for 'easy'. Realistic, in this case, means 'do-able'. It is important to devise a plan or a way of getting there which makes the goal realistic for you. Do not set goals too high or too low. When goals are set unrealistically high they are perceived to be unreachable and no effort will be made to achieve them. Conversely goals can be set so low that you feel no challenge or benefit in achieving them. Therefore always set goals that are challenging, but realistic.

Timely goals

Without careful thought and planning, goal setting can be unsystematic, sporadic and disorganised. In this case goals will be forgotten, achievement of goals will not be measured and feedback will not be incorporated in developing new goals. The major benefits of goal setting will therefore have been lost. Be organised and methodical in the way that you use goal setting simply by setting a timeframe for the goal. For example, complete by next week, in three months or by the end of term. This identifies an end point to your goal and gives you a clear target to work towards. If you fail to set a time, the commitment is too vague. It tends not to happen because you feel you can start at any time. Without a time limit, there is no urgency to start taking action now. In addition, too many un-prioritised goals may be set, leading to a feeling of overload. Remember that you also need to plan social time in order to relax.

It should be noted that when setting goals you should consider the experiential taxonomy that has been utilised within the programme of study. A specified level might be required within that assessment strategy to be awarded a pass. For example, if using the Benner (1984) model, you may have to achieve a level of competence. If Steinaker and Bell's (1979) model is used, you may have to achieve a level of internalisation. An awareness of which level you will be expected to achieve will be required when setting your goals so that you know what to aim for.

Action planning

Once a goal or goals have been set, it is necessary to look at how to achieve them. Action planning typically includes deciding what you are going to do, how you are going to do it, by when and in what order so you have a clear, structured plan to reach your goals. All too often limited plans are produced which lack detail of how the goal will be achieved; nevertheless, with encouragement you can develop a detailed plan that is realistic, feasible, and likely to succeed. Many action plans fail because the tasks appear too difficult, or they may have several goals. However they can still be achievable. Whatever your goals, whatever stage you are at in the decision making process, you are most likely to make progress and succeed if you break down the tasks you have to do into small steps and then identify the actions you need to take for each step. Set a timescale for each action – but be realistic – do not expect the impossible. Action planning does require adequate time as a process to develop learning, but if used effectively, it can be a powerful tool for self-management and achievement of identified goals.

When writing your action plan and identify a range of ways of tackling your goals, the next step is to help identify those strategies which best fit your learning style and situation. Also try to identify those factors which might help or hinder successful resolution and at this point referring to your SWOT analysis will become essential as you will have previously identified those factors. Some factors will be more powerful than others and it might be useful for you to underline those factors that will most strongly influence movement towards or away from your goals, as these will certainly influence your action plan. Nicklin and Kenworthy (2000) suggest that an action plan is concerned with maximising those factors that will help you progress to your goals and minimising or neutralising factors that will hinder progress.

An example of an action plan is shown in *Figure 2.1*. You will note that the outcome goals and performance goals relate to the information given in previous examples (see *Tables 2.2 and 2.3*). The outcome goal only relates to achieving part of outcome level 2 as the purpose of this is to apply the principle of SMART thus focusing on the assessment stage so it is manageable and achievable. The same process will need to be repeated for planning and delivering care outlined in the other parts of learning outcome level 2 (see *Table 2.2*).

Mentorship and supervision

The portfolio approach, as previously suggested, is more directed towards a student-led approach focusing on experiential learning. This will predominantly take place in the clinical setting under the direction and supervision of an appropriately qualified practitioner who is often referred to as a mentor. The term supervision is used in a general sense to describe the role someone has in overseeing the work of another (Quinn, 2000). Supervision has also been applied to the term mentorship and has therefore been implied in the description and role of a mentor.

The concept of mentoring and supervision in nurse education is not a new one. The origins of mentoring began in the United States and started to appear in the nursing literature in the early 1980s, followed by a wealth of published literature in the 1990s (Andrews and Wallis, 1999). Although mentorship has assumed respectability in professional education, it remains a term that is not easily defined due to the terminology frequently used to describe a mentor. These include 'preceptor', 'supervisor', 'coach', 'facilitator', 'assessor' and 'teacher' which are sometimes used synonymously (Darling, 1985; Jarvis and Gibson, 1997; Neary, 1997; Chow and Suen, 2001). Despite substantial variations in the meanings of these terms (Hughes, 2004) the frequent use of different terminologies has caused confusion of definitions and roles due to diverse contexts in which mentorship functions (Phillips, 1994). It is however beyond the scope of this chapter to debate the various terminologies used, so taking a simplistic view a mentor, as defined by the English National Board (1997) is

an appropriately qualified and experience first level nurse/midwife/health visitor who, by example and facilitation, guides, assists and supports the student's learning.

A mentor should be able to support your learning and assessment of clinical practice against the required Nursing and Midwifery Council (2006) standards. This applies whether you are a pre-registration nursing student, midwifery student, or seeking to gain a specialist practice qualification (SPQ) that is recordable on the nurses' part of the register, or a registerable advanced nursing practice (ANP) qualification. However, from 2008, SPQ and ANP students will be required to have support and be assessed by a practice teacher (Nursing and Midwifery Council, 2006).

Mentors may also be required for other continuing professional development modules and programmes of study which are not recorded or registered with the Nursing and Midwifery Council, and they may still be responsible for assessing practice and competence.

Benner (1984) recommends that the role of the mentor in clinical practice is to facilitate the transition from novice to competent practitioner. This means that the role of the mentor should include a number of functions to enable you to work together to achieve the desired outcomes. The Nursing and Midwifery Council (2006: 30) has set standards for the role and suggests that the mentor should

Table 2.4. Role of mentor and student at different levels of experiential taxonomies

Taxonomic level (Steinaker and Bell)	Taxonomic level (Benner)	Role of the mentor/teacher	Role of the student
Exposure	Novice	Motivator Information provider Coach Role model	Attender
Participation	Advanced beginner	Catalyst Coach Role model	Explorer
Identification	Competent	Moderator Coach Role model	Experimenter
Internalisation	Proficient	Sustainer Coach Role model	Extender
Dissemination	Expert	Critic and evaluator Coach Role model	Influencer

■ Provide support and guidance to you (as the student) when learning new skills or applying new knowledge.
■ Act as a resource to you to facilitate your learning and professional growth.
■ Directly manage your learning in practice to ensure public protection.
■ Directly observe your practice, or use indirect observation where appropriate, in order to ensure defined outcomes and competencies are met.

In the early stages of the relationship you may initially appear dependent or reliant on your mentor in terms of the intensity of the support offered. This is necessary as you begin your learning journey through the experiential taxonomic levels. As your relationship, clinical experience and movement through the hierarchical levels of the experiential taxonomies develops, your needs and priorities will change. As a result your role as a student and the role of your mentor will change (Morton-Cooper and Palmer, 2000). This is illustrated in *Table 2.4* using Steinaker and Bell's (1979) and Benner's (1984) experiential taxonomies.

Mentorship is seen by many writers as being a long-term relationship that extends throughout a student's programme, whereas others limit it to the concept of a relationship within a specific placement. In some systems, classical mentoring (George and Kummerow, 1981) is advocated, where students are encouraged to choose their own mentors. In others, contract mentoring is suggested (Morton-Cooper and Palmer, 2000), where an artificial relationship is created for a specific purpose, hence a mentor is assigned to the student. The former is preferable if possible as this increases the likelihood of compatibility between the student and mentor which is an important factor in the relationship. This is because the student and mentor may be drawn together naturally by their personal characteristics, attributes and common values and thus develop a mutual and trusting relationship. However, the 'assigned mentor' is the more likely model to be adopted within pre-registration and many other Nursing and Midwifery Council approved programmes of study, where employing authorities need to allocate appropriately qualified staff to fulfil the role of mentor.

Personal qualities are also central to the success of the mentorship process, as a partnership should be based on mutual trust and respect. Darling (1984) identifies some personal qualities that she considers to be the absolute requirements for a significant mentoring relationship. These are:

- *Attraction*: The student admires and desires to emulate the mentor.
- *Action*: The mentor invests time and energy in teaching, guiding and helping the student.
- *Affection*: The mentor demonstrates respect, encouragement and support for the student.

At the initial meeting with your mentor you should discuss what your expectations from each other are, what you hope to gain from your learning experience and relationship, the outcomes you need to achieve, your SWOT analysis, your goals and action plan. Your mentor will be able to provide information, guidance, support and constructive feedback as to whether the goals you have set and your action plans are realistic and achievable. This is important as this information can be used to set ground rules and develop a learning contract so that the student and mentor are committed to developing an effective, successful relationship to facilitate the learning experience to achieve outcomes.

Setting ground rules

Ground rules are simply statements of values and guidelines that will facilitate the process of learning. They help to create a safe and effective learning environment based on mutual trust and respect through an established, mutually

Table 2.5. Issues to consider prior to writing ground rules

- Recognise that a mentoring relationship is voluntary
- Identify your expectations clearly
- Identify your mentor's availability and frequency of meetings
- Identify other roles/workload of your mentor
- Ensure you are both actively involved
- Identify how frequently you will evaluate and renew your relationship
- Identify confidentiality issues
- Develop and work to a written learning contract

Table 2.6. Common ground rules

- Treat each other with respect, even in the face of disagreement
- Develop a personal relationship to enhance trust and open communication
- Have a shared understanding of learning needs and development
- Work together for a minimum of two shifts per week
- Do not make excessive demands on each other's time and negotiate a system for the best use of time
- Arrange weekly meetings to discuss progress
- Arrive on time for scheduled meetings
- Ensure that feedback is constructive
- Respect each other's privacy
- Evaluate the relationship every four weeks

agreed set of expectations and behaviours; thus preventing misunderstandings and disagreements. To be effective, ground rules must be clear, consistent, agreed-to, and followed. Each partnership varies and therefore creates its own ground rules. In addition, ground rules that govern the working relationship will also vary according to the needs of the student and mentor and should therefore be reviewed and renewed periodically.

The student and mentor will have some clear ideas of what they want beforehand. There are some issues that may need to be considered and these may be succinct or exhaustive depending on a variety of factors. *Table 2.5* gives some examples of common issues to consider when determining ground rules and *Table 2.6* gives examples of ground rules that may be utilised.

As previously stated the issues to consider prior to developing ground rules may be succinct or exhaustive, this equally applies to ground rules depending on the student and the mentor's expectations, and the learning needs and development at that particular time. It is important to note that however extensive the ground rules may be, it is advisable to reduce their number to keep them to a workable agreement so all rules can be realistically adhered to. Remember that the working relationship may change and consequently the ground rules may change.

Learning contracts

The UKCC *Fitness for Practice* (1999: 38) recommendation 13 states:

> *Students, assessors and mentors should know what is expected of them through specified practice outcomes which form part of a formal learning contract.*

Learning contracts can, if carefully negotiated between the student and mentor fulfil this recommendation as it is a negotiated signed agreement that specifies aims, learning objectives and outcomes to be accomplished, resources which can be used, criteria and methods for evaluation and final assessment procedures (Neary, 2000). In addition, learning contracts are flexible and can provide a great deal of autonomy and independence in learning (Brown and Knight, 1994). Learning contracts can be simple or as complex as the learning and assessment strategy requires, with various types of learning contracts utilised for different purposes, eg. for programmes of study, practice placements, distance learning. Whatever the type and format, they should be a signed mutual agreement between the student and mentor to structure the learning experience.

Details should include:

- What you need to learn/be able to do (learning or placement objectives).
- How you will go about learning, ie. who and what will help (strategies and resources to achieve objectives).
- What you can produce to show that learning has been successful (evidence to indicate achievement of objectives.
- How and by whom the learning will be assessed (criteria for evaluating the evidence).

Figure 2.2 gives an example of how this information is presented in a learning contract in relation to the learning outcomes in *Table 2.2*. These can also be used as evidence within your portfolio, which will demonstrate the process of how you have progressed through the stages of experiential taxonomies.

Personal Learning Contract – Proposal Form
Student's name: .... Mentor's name: ....
Date agreed: .... Date for review: ....

What incident or event makes you think about what you will need to learn?	Learning Objectives (what you need to achieve/learn)	Strategies and resources (what you intend to do and what facilities you need to achieve objectives)	What is to be reviewed/assessed (The evidence you will produce to show that you have met your objectives)	Criteria for review/assessment (what will demonstrate that you have been successful)	Timescale (when you intend to have completed this piece of learning)
Having observed staff nurses perform comprehensive clinical assessment, apply interventions based on national guidelines to patients with acute exacerbation of asthma, I recognised that knowledge and skills are very limited in relation to assessment of respiratory problems, pathophysiology of respiratory diseases and appropriate interventions	Demonstrate the ability to assess, plan and deliver care that is responsive, flexible, relevant and effective in relation to a patient with an acute exacerbation of asthma to a competent level	To work closely with my mentor and to observe, participate and question to increase my knowledge, skills and understanding. To review anatomy, physiology and pathophysiology. Talk to patients to understand their experience of the disease. To review national and local guidelines to increase my knowledge of interventions and appropriate treatment	My competence in assessing, planning and implementing appropriate timely care to patients with an acute exacerbation of asthma. Reflective journal of my learning. Personal reflection and analysis based on a case study of a patient presenting with this condition	Positive comments and evaluation from my mentor. Evaluation of patient's care to assess effectiveness of care. Patients' comments and reactions. My own confidence in assessing, planning and implementing care. Successfully completing module	3 months initially, but can be viewed as ongoing development to continue to improve

Signature of student: Signature of mentor:

Figure 2.2. *Example of a learning contract adapted from Challis (2000) contract design.*

Summary

In summary, assessment is a vital part of the educational process and portfolios, as an educational assessment strategy, are viewed as a valuable tool for measuring the quality, quantity, progress and achievement of learning, particularly in the direction of experiential learning. In addition, it helps the student to become an active participant during the learning experience, through the use of self-assessment tools such as SWOT analysis, goal setting and action planning. As learning from experience takes place predominantly in the workplace, the student's relationship with the mentor is very important in supporting, encouraging and promoting growth and development to successfully achieve outcomes. The utilisation of the aforementioned learning tools can be constructive and worthwhile to ensure an effective, successful learning journey in producing a portfolio for assessment.

References

Andrews M, Wallis M (1999) Mentorship in nursing: A literature review. *J Adv Nursing* **29**(1): 201–07

Bandura A (1997) *Self-efficacy: The Exercise of Control.* Freeman, New York

Baume D (2001) *A Briefing on Assessment and Portfolios Assessment Series No 6.* Learning and Teaching Support Network, York

Benner P (1984) *From Novice to Expert. Excellence and Power in Clinical Nursing Practice.* Addison-Wesley Publishing, Menlo Park, California

Bloom BS (1956) *Taxonomy of Educational Objectives: The Classification of Educational Goals, Handbook I: Cognitive Domain.* David McKay Inc, New York

Bloom BS, Krathwohl DR, Masia BB (1964) *A Handbook of Educational Objectives. Handbook II: The Affective Domain.* David McKay Inc, New York

Boud D (1990) Assessment and the promotion of academic values. *Studies in Higher Education* **15**(1): 101–11

Boud D (1992) The use of self-assessment schedule in negotiated learning. *Studies in Higher Education* **17**(2): 85–200

Boud D (1995) *Enhancing Learning Through Self Assessment.* Routledge, London

Brown RA (1992) *Portfolio Development and Profiling for Nurses.* Quay Publishing, Lancaster

Brown S, Knight P (1994) *Assessing Learners in Higher Education.* Kogan Page, London

Challis M (2000) AMEE Medical Education Guide No. 19: Personal learning plans. *Medical Teacher* **22**: 225–36

Chow FLW, Suen LKP (2001) Clinical staff as mentors in pre-registration undergraduate nursing education: Students' perceptions of the mentors' roles and responsibilities. *Nurse Education Today* **21**: 350–8

Confucius (551BC-479BC) Confucius Quotes – the Quotations Page. From: www. quotationspage.com/quotes/confucius [Accessed 22 November 2006]

Darling LAW (1984) What do nurses want in a mentor? *Nurse Educator* **11**(2): 42–4

Darling L (1985) Mentors and mentoring. *Nurse Educator* **10**(6): 18–19

Dewey J (1938) *Experience and Education.* Collier, New York

Downie CM, Basford P (1997) *Teaching and Assessing in Clinical Practice. A Reader.* University of Greenwich, London

Dreyfus SE (1982) Formal models vs. human situational understanding:Inherent limitations on the modelling of business expertise. *Office: Technology and People* **1**: 133–55

Dreyfus HL, Dreyfus SE (1980). The Dreyfus Model of Skill Acquisition applied to nursing. In Benner P (ed) From Novice to Expert In Benner P (ed) *From Novice to Expert. Excellence and Power in Clinical Nursing Practice.* Addison-Wesley Publishing, Menlo Park, California

English National Board (1997) *Standards for Approval of Higher Education Institutions and Programmes.* English National Board, London

Frith DS, Macintosh HG (1984) *A Teacher's Guide to Self-assessment.* Stanley Thornes, Cheltenham

George P, Kummerow J (1981) Mentoring for career women. *Training* **18**(2): 44–9

Harrow AJ (1972) *Taxonomy of Psychomotor Domain: A Guide for Developing Behavioural Objectives.* David McKay Inc, New York

Higher Education Quality Control (1996) *Guidelines on Quality Assurance.* HEQC, London

Hughes SJ (2004) The mentoring role of the personal tutor in the 'Fitness for practice' curriculum: An all Wales approach. *Nurse Education in Practice* **4**: 271–8

Jarvis P, Gibson S (1997) *The Teacher Practitioner and Mentor in Nursing, Midwifery, Health Visiting and the Social Services.* (2nd edn) Routledge, London

Kolb DA (1984) *Experiential Learning: Experience as the Source of Learning and Development.* Prentice Hall, Englewood Cliffs

Latham CL, Fahey LJ (2006) Novice to expert advanced practice nurse role transition: Guided student. *Journal of Nursing Education* **45**(1): 46–8

Locke EA, Latham GP (1990) *A Theory of Goal Setting and Task Performance.* Prentice Hall, Englewood Cliffs

Moon J (2002) *The Module and Programme Development Handbook.* Kogan Page, London

Morton-Cooper A, Palmer A (2000) *Mentorship, Preceptorship and Clinical Supervision. A Guide to Professional Support Roles in Clinical Practice.* (2nd edn.) Blackwell Science, Oxford

Neary M (1997) Defining the role of assessors, mentors and supervisors: Part 2.

Nursing Standard **11**(43): 34–8

Neary M (2000) *Teaching, Assessing and Evaluation for Clinical Competence. A Practice Guide for Practitioners and Teachers.* Stanley Thornes. Cheltenham.

Nicklin P, Kenworthy N (1995) *Teaching and Assessing in Nursing Practice* (2nd edn) Scutari Press, London

Nicklin P, Kenworthy N (2000) *Teaching and Assessing in Nursing Practice. An Experiential approach.* (3rd edn.) Balliere Tindall, London

Nursing and Midwifery Council (2006a) *The PREP Handbook.* Nursing and Midwifery Council, London

Nursing and Midwifery Council (2006b) *Standards to Support Learning and Assessment in Practice. NMC Standards for Mentors, Practice Teachers and Teachers.* Nursing and Midwifery Council, London

Phillips R (1994) Providing student support systems in Project 2000 nurse education programmes – the personal tutor role of nurse teachers. *Nurse Education Today* **14**: 216–222

Quinn FM (1998) Reflection and reflective practice. In Quinn FM, Humphries J (eds) *Continuing Professional Development in Nursing. A Handbook for Practitioners and Educators.* Stanley Thorpes, Cheltenham

Quinn FM (2000) *Principles and Practice of Nurse Education.* (4th edn) Stanley Thornes Ltd, Cheltenham

Redfern E (1998) The power of the professional profile. In Quinn FM, Humphries J (eds) *Continuing Professional Development in Nursing: A Guide for Practitioners and Educators.* Stanley Thornes, Cheltenham

Rowntree D (1977) *Assessing Students: How Shall We Know Them?* Harper and Rowe, London

Scholes J, Webb C, Gray M, Endacott R, Miller C, Jasper M, McMullen M (2004) Making portfolios work in practice. *J Adv Nursing* **46**(6): 595–603

Schunk DH (2001) *Self-Regulation Through Goal Setting.* From: www. tourettesyndrome.net [accessed 20th December 2006]

Simpson E (1966) *The Classification of Educational Objectives, Psychomotor Domain.* University of Illinois Press, Illinois

Steinaker NW, Bell MR (1979) *The Experiential Taxonomy. A New Approach to Teaching and Learning.* Academic Press, London

United Kingdom Central Council (1999) *Fitness for Practice.* UKCC, London

Webster M, Guralnik DB (1976) *Webster's New World Dictionary of the American Language* (2nd edn) William Collins and World Publishing Company, Ohio

Zimmerman BJ (1998) Developing self-fulfilling cycles of academic regulation: An analysis of exemplary instructional models. In Schunk DH, Zimmerman BJ (eds) *Self-regulated Learning: From Teaching to Self-reflective Practice.* Guilford Press, New York

CHAPTER 3

Providing evidence of achievement

Kay Norman

Introduction

This chapter discusses many types of evidence that may be used within a portfolio. However, this is not an exhaustive list, and it is hoped that students will be creative and innovative in devising ways of producing the required evidence necessary in order to complete their portfolios.

Good preparation is the key to a successful portfolio. Portfolios are a personal account of learning, and therefore it is important that students feel comfortable with the chosen methods. However they can be seen as a tool to provide critical reflection of a learning journey, and therefore exploring the many varieties of evidence available to use will add to the student's body of knowledge for future development. Examples of the types of evidence that may be utilised are included, as is a discussion on reflective writing and presentation skills.

There are numerous forms of evidence that may be submitted within a portfolio, however these will differ greatly depending on their required function.

The evidence within a portfolio will enable an assessor to measure student learning, and enable a student to show progression throughout a period of time/ study, provide critical reflections of situations and incidents that are pertinent to the student's learning, demonstrate self-directed learning, provide details of competence within required learning outcomes, and capture the student's learning journey of personal and professional development.

As already discussed, portfolios in the nursing profession have many uses, and therefore it is imperative that you take time to ascertain all relevant information and necessary requirements prior to commencement.

A portfolio to be completed as an assessment for a postgraduate 30 credit module in nursing leadership will have a different format and content to a portfolio required as part of a pre-registration nursing diploma programme.

When compiling a portfolio, it is important to ask the questions why, what and who to ensure that the content and format meet the necessary requirements.

- Why are you compiling the portfolio?

- As part of an ongoing assessment (such as during pre-registration nurse training).
- For continuing professional development.
- As assessment of a module/course of study.
- For APEL (Accreditation of Prior Experiential Learning).

■ What evidence do I need to include?
- Are there learning outcomes to be achieved, if so what is the academic level required (eg. diploma, undergraduate, postgraduate)?
- Are there guidelines on types of evidence to be included?
- Are there specific section headings that must be included?
- Is there a word limit imposed (minimum and maximum)?

■ Who will be reading the portfolio?
- Course/module leader if part of an assessment.
- Nursing and Midwifery Council/you for your own personal/ professional development as part of PREP (Post-registration Education and Practice).
- Potential employers.
- Assessment panels (regarding APEL applications).
- Mentor/supervisor.

Table 3.1. Timetable in preparation of an assessed portfolio

Date	Activity	Resulting action
September	Plan structure, revisit learning outcomes required, check understanding of components	Plan section headings, formulate action plans for each outcome. Discuss with supervisor
October	Commence learning diary and plan learning visits	Read around models of reflection
November	Write reflections on case studies/critical incidents	Revisit action plans. Gather testimonials/witness statements
December	Reflect on study days and visits with specialist nurses. Present to practice team	Organise cross-referencing system. Ensure robust index system
January	Complete reflections and all methods of evidence required. Documentation to be dated and signed as necessary	Ask colleague to proofread. Ensure all elements required are included

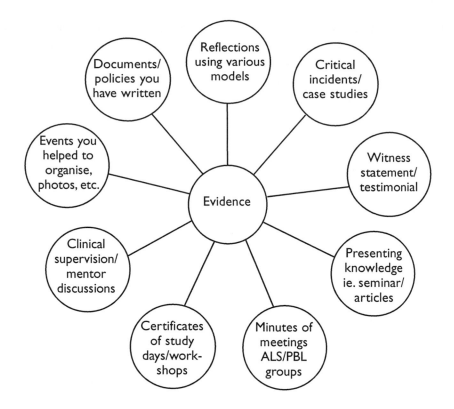

Figure 3.1. Types of evidence. ALS: action learning sets; PBL: problem-based learning.

If there is a time frame involved, it may be useful to plan a timetable to give structure and direction to activities. Allow plenty of time to gather and write the evidence required, and also time to organise and cross reference this within the portfolio. *Table 3.1* is an example of a timetable for a portfolio which forms part of a module assessment.

Figure 3.1 gives examples of evidence that could be included within a portfolio, it does not mean that all of these elements need to, or should be included. Certain types of evidence will be discussed in more detail to give further explanations and insights into how these can be used effectively within your portfolio.

Reflections can be included alongside any of the methods of evidence. For example, you may wish to include a critical incident form (maintaining anonymity of the people/placement involved), a reflective piece of writing analysing what you have learnt from the situation, the risk assessment strategy, how you will link this to improving your own practice, and an action plan in order to reduce the situation occurring again.

There may be a policy or protocol you have been involved in formulating or renewing. This could be submitted as part of a reflection that considers the issues arising from implementing the policy, such as management support, collaborating with colleagues, any barriers that occurred, national/local directives adhered to, dissemination of good practice, etc.

Reflection

The concept of reflection is a key component of transformative learning theory (Cranton, 1994; Mezirow 1998). The original idea of this appears to stem from Dewey (1938) who defined reflection as

active, persistent and careful consideration of any belief or supposed form of knowledge in the light of the grounds that support it, and the further conclusion to which it tends.

Within professional practice, the work of Schon (1987) has been instrumental in promoting the application of scientific theory in making decisions and problem solving through reflective practice.

The degree to which reflective practice has been adopted by the nursing profession is significant, with professional bodies such as the Nursing and Midwifery Council (NMC) reaffirming support for the concept of the reflective practitioner. It appears to be inherent in all accredited nursing programmes at all academic levels, and even those that are not often have an element of reflection. For example, a workshop delivered by a healthcare trust may require, as part of the evaluation, group members to reflect on how this will change their practice, what they will do differently and how they felt about the discussions and content of the day.

However, within the nursing profession, there is a distinct difference between 'thoughtful practice' and 'reflective practice'. Jarvis (1992) suggests that the reflective practitioner is one who is able to problematise many situations of professional performance so that they can become potential learning situations. It is this emphasis on learning that has encouraged the inclusion of reflective practice into nursing education programmes (Hannigan, 2001).

Content and process reflection allows professional nurses to synthesise, predict and evaluate while considering context and accessing professional knowledge and experience. Such reflection can occur before (anticipatory reflection), during (reflection in action) and after (reflection on action) practice (Saylor, 1990; Van Manen, 1991).

In order to embrace reflective practice, you must want to practise to the best of your ability, be motivated to continually improve personal and professional practice, and be open minded to new ways of thinking. This will lead to self-confidence in challenging assumptions, new information, knowledge, understanding and insight (Teekman, 2000). Support from your mentor, supervisor, educational tutors and peers will help to encourage this process.

It is not the aim of this book to delve into the many theoretical writings on reflective practice. However, this will be an important area within your portfolio and therefore examples of reflective models or frameworks that you may wish to use to structure your reflections will be explored.

Ascertain at what academic level your reflective writing will be. This will need to be established prior to commencement, as an assessor will be marking reflective writing to the criteria for that particular level, eg. undergraduate criteria will be different from postgraduate criteria. In order to show analysis and critical thinking, references to appropriate literature will need to be included to support your discussions and points raised.

Many students ask how long a piece of reflection should be. This is impossible to answer, but it is important if the reflection is part of an assessment, that the minimum and maximum word limit is adhered to if specified. If not, you have control. Remember, the reflection should primarily be about learning, moving practice forward, analysing situations in order to highlight areas for improvement, and to show personal and professional progression.

The model of reflection you choose may determine the depth of information you feel able to discuss and analyse about a certain situation. However, it may not be apparent that learning and analysis of thoughts and ideas has taken place if only a few lines are written.

Many students feel able to write more on the descriptive components of reflective writing, eg. 'what happened', but find it difficult to explore in depth a 'feelings' section of a reflective model. If a model is used correctly, there should be sufficient coverage of all the issues needed. You may want to use the sub-headings of the varying models to structure your writing.

As you continue to use varying models, you will become more confident in exploring the areas required. When you feel confident in reflective writing, you may wish to structure your writing without adhering to a rigid framework of a reflective model, but introduce your reflection as 'based on elements of Johns' model of reflection' (see below). This may be beneficial in case studies where areas outside the normal reflective framework need to be discussed and analysed, or where you feel sub-headings of the model detract from the context of your writing.

You may want to generate a 'reflection group' among your fellow students. It is sometimes easier knowing that there are others who are experiencing the same kinds of difficulties and concerns with reflective writing, and you can also gain inspiration from those who have mastered the process. This also helps in discussing varying models that have been used, and how analysis of issues has been included. Ground rules are a must for these groups and need to be agreed by all members, in order that learning and inclusion remains the focus.

Table 3.2. Example of reflective structure for a study day/workshop

Title of study day/date/time
- What were my aims/expectations of the day?
- Were these fully met, if not why?
- What have I learned as a result of this day?
- How will I incorporate this learning into practice?
- How will I disseminate this knowledge to others?

When accessing relevant literature in order to inform your analysis, it is important that the wider literature is used to inform your reflection, do not concentrate solely on searches for specific research related to your situation as this may prove sparse. In the example below there may not be much literature specifically relating to student nurses' experiences on medical wards.

You are reflecting on an incident where you felt uncomfortable and anxious while on a medical ward placement, due to lack of support from staff. You felt unable to ask for further opportunities to learn relevant procedures as everyone always seemed too busy. Your mentor was on annual leave, and you had not been allocated a member of staff to work with. You were the only nursing student on that particular ward.

From the above situation, to inform your knowledge base in order to analyse the various issues arising, you may want to look at literature on teamwork, communication, assertiveness, collaboration, and self-awareness. This will encourage a more in depth learning experience and will support a wider understanding of the issues involved.

If the reflection is to support further evidence such as a study day attended, it may be sufficient to write a brief reflection as an evaluation on what you have learnt from the day. See *Table 3.2* for an example of a reflective structure. A model of reflection may not always be needed in this instance. Related literature may still be used in the analysis of issues if required and relevant.

The following are some examples of reflective models and frameworks that you may wish to use within your portfolio to structure your reflective writing. There are many others available which are not included in this book that you may want to explore. It is advisable to use a variety of models/frameworks within your portfolio to show how you have broadened your learning around reflection, and introduce why you have chosen a particular model, ie. because of its ease of use, because sections of the model related well to your scenario, because the framework gave a logical structure to your writing, or because the model gave a broader scope to reflect on wider issues, etc.

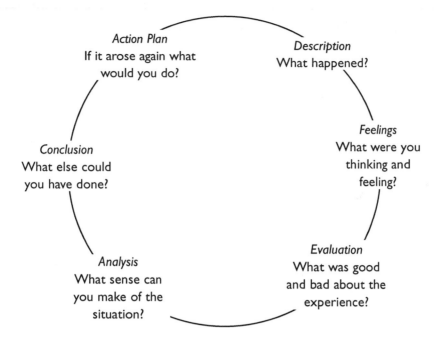

Figure 3.2. Gibbs' (1988) reflective cycle.

Gibbs' reflective cycle

Gibbs (1988) reflective cycle (see *Figure 3.2*) is a framework that encourages a clear description of the situation, analysis of feelings, evaluation of the experience, and analysis to make sense of the experience. The conclusion component is where other options can be considered, reflecting on the experience to help think about what you would do if the situation arose again. It is similar to Kolb's learning cycle in that it is arranged in a circular format, and the cues are quite general and less prescriptive than other, more directive models.

This cycle is fairly straightforward to use, and can be used to structure your reflective writing. However, if you are using it to structure your writing at undergraduate or postgraduate levels you may need to adjust the cycle so that analysis permeates throughout each stage.

Johns' model and Rolfe et al's framework

Johns' (2000) model for structured reflection (see *Table 3.3*) can be used as a guide for analysis of a critical incident or general reflection on experience. This can be useful for more complex decision making and analysis. Johns supports the need for learners to work with a supervisor throughout their learning experience with Rolfe *et al* (2001) describing the model as a facilitator's

Table 3.3. Johns' model for structured reflection

Reflective clue	Way of knowing
• Bring the mind home	
• Focus on a description of an experience that seems significant in some way	Aesthetics
• What particular issues seem significant to pay attention to?	Aesthetics
• How were others feeling and what made me feel that way?	Aesthetics
• How was I feeling and what made me feel that way?	Personal
• What was I trying to achieve and did I respond effectively?	Aesthetics
• What were the consequences of my actions on the patient, others and myself?	Aesthetics
• What factors influenced the way I was feeling, thinking or responding?	Personal
• What knowledge did or might have informed me?	Empirics
• To what extent did I act for the best and in tune with my values?	Ethics
• How does this situation connect with previous experiences?	Reflexivity
• How might I respond more effectively given this situation again?	Reflexivity
• What would be the consequences of alternative actions for the patient, others and myself?	Reflexivity
• How do I feel *now* about this experience?	Reflexivity
• Am I able to support myself and others better as a consequence?	Reflexivity
• Am I more able to realise desirable practice monitored using appropriate frameworks such as framing perspectives, Carper's fundamental ways of knowing, other maps?	Reflexivity

framework for reflection. Johns refers to this as guided reflection, and recommends that students use a structured diary. Johns considered that through sharing reflections on learning experiences greater understanding of those experiences could be achieved than by reflection as a lone exercise. Johns' influences can be seen in Carper's (1978) four patterns of knowing, aesthetics, personal ethics, and empirics, adding a fifth pattern 'reflexivity'.

Table 3.4. Rolfe *et al*'s framework for reflexive practice

Descriptive level of reflection	Theory- and knowledge-building level of reflection	Action-orientated (reflexive) level of reflection
What	*So what*	*Now what*
• is the problem/ difficulty/reason for being stuck/reason for feeling bad/reason we don't get on, etc.?	• does this tell me/teach me/imply/mean about me/my patient/others/ our relationship/my patient's care/the model of care I am using/my attitudes/my patient's attitudes/etc.	• do I need to do in order to make things better/stop being stuck/improve my patient's care/resolve the situation/feel better/ get on better/etc.?
• was my role in the situation?		• broader issues need to be considered if this action is to be successful?
• was I trying to achieve?	• was going through my mind as I acted?	
• actions did I take?		
• was the response of others?	• did I base my actions on?	• might be the consequences of this action?
• were the consequences for the patient? for myself? for others?	• other knowledge can I bring to the situation? experiential personal scientific	
• feelings did it evoke in the patient? in myself? in others?	• could/should I have done to make it better?	
• was good/bad about the experience?	• is my new understanding of the situation?	
	• broader issues arise from the situation?	

Rolfe *et al* (2001) suggests however, that if the situation remained ongoing, the practitioner would want to know, 'How can I take this forward?' They do not consider that Johns has made provision for this question. If you use this model for a situation that is ongoing you would need to review and adapt the reflexive section using stages/suggestions from another model or develop your own set of cues.

Rolfe *et al* (2001) propose a reflexive framework (see *Table 3.4*) that is based on Borton's (1970) simple developmental model. The questions, what, so what, and now what can stimulate reflection and the framework is suggested for use by advanced practitioners. However, it is a simple and easy to understand framework of reflection and would be beneficial at all levels of practice. The framework has a sequential and cyclical order. First, the practitioner reflects on the situation in order to describe it. Second, the practitioner is encouraged to construct personal theory and knowledge about the situation in order to learn from it. At the third level the practitioner reflects on action and considers ways of improving the situation and reflects on the consequences of his or her actions. Rolfe *et al* (2001) consider this final stage as the one that can make the greatest contribution to practice.

Atkins and Murphy's model of reflection

Atkins and Murphy's (1994) model (*Figure 3.3*) sets out specific stages to structure reflective writing and can be useful when reflecting on critical incidents or case studies. Unfortunately the first stage of this model suggests that reflection in nursing is often stimulated by uncomfortable thoughts and feelings, which has resulted in many students thinking that reflection is primarily concerned with negative situations. This is certainly not the aim of reflection, where positive situations can be reflected upon to disseminate good practice, act as a basis to improve practice further, and ultimately learn from that experience.

Throughout the portfolio, you may wish to reflect on many situations including case studies, critical incidents, teaching sessions, presentations, meetings attended, action learning sets and problem-based learning scenarios.

Therefore it is important that you take time to understand and appreciate the benefit of reflection. It may be appropriate within your portfolio to write more than one reflection concerning the same scenario.

You are helping to dress a leg ulcer on Mrs X with your community nurse mentor. Mrs X appears withdrawn and upset, and you ask her if she is ok as this is the first time you have met her. She explains that her husband passed away 12 months ago, and she has felt depressed ever since. She has no family nearby and feels isolated and lonely. The community nurse caseload for the day is overbooked and you are already 30 minutes behind schedule for visits. Your mentor advises Mrs X that she will ensure her GP is informed and will ask for a home visit request to ascertain all relevant issues and concerns, but she must leave in order to attend to her next patient. You feel frustrated and angry that you could not spend more time with Mrs X to try to allay her worries and fears.

You may wish to write an initial reflection on the situation utilising Gibbs' model to describe what happened and how you felt at the time. You may also wish to read the wider literature around the political healthcare agenda,

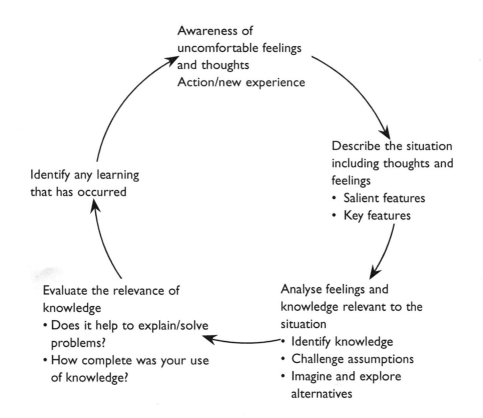

Figure 3.3. Atkins and Murphy's model of reflection.

communication, roles of primary care staff and community nursing, patient expectations and what the general public expects from nurses, in order to inform your analysis of the situation.

From this, an action plan can be developed to help you prepare a strategy if the situation arose again. On the following visits to Mrs X, you may have decided to discuss your reflection with your mentor, discussing the constraints of primary care staff, collaborative working with other colleagues such as the community mental health team, leadership, and resources of services. You may want to discuss the suggestions of the GP, whether sufficient time can be planned within the visit to ensure appropriate discussions take place with Mrs X, whether social services should be involved, or whether there are local voluntary services available to incorporate social activities, such as visits to day centres, etc.

Following these discussions and implementation of any initiatives, another reflection may be of use to show how the situation has improved or changed and what positive aspects or barriers occurred in the process. This will show progression of your learning journey and demonstrate your understanding of the reflective process as a continual cycle.

Learning outcome context	Areas to be observed	Designation and signature of observer	Date observed/ comments of observer
To understand and demonstrate principles of screening within a health care context	Communication skills		
	History taking		
New patient health check within a primary health care centre	Understanding the importance of family history		
	Correct use of screening equipment ie. BP, weight, height, BMI		
	To know when and who to refer to as required		
	Demonstrate principles of screening to the patient population		

Figure 3.4. Example of a witness statement.

It is important to note that any previous work that has been summatively assessed cannot be included within a portfolio if it forms part of the evidence required for assessment purposes, ie. a piece of work cannot be assessed twice.

Testimonials and witness statements

Within your portfolio there will be instances when you will be observed in practice. This may be through your mentor or another specified colleague observing a skill, presentation, general working practice, specific management of a patient, consultation and history taking skills, and any other area of practice deemed necessary in order to progress or improve practice and/or to achieve learning-related outcomes.

As part of the evidence you provide within your portfolio, these observations should be recorded, signed and dated by the observer (see *Figures 3.4 and 3.5*). Some observers may wish to write a report or statement in detail concerning the observations made, others may not be in a position to write such an in depth summary. It is important before the observation commences, that you and the observer discuss how the session is to be documented and what learning

Area visited: ....

Date of visit: ....Time: From .... To ....

General aim of visit:

....

....

....

....

Objectives of visit

1. ....

2. ....

3. ....

4. ....

5. ....

Signed (name and designation): ....Date ....

Comments: ....

....

....

....

....

Figure 3.5. Example of a witness statement template for a practice visit.

outcomes are to be addressed. A pre-written form can be negotiated prior to the observation to set direction for both yourself and the observer in order to focus on the areas required. If the observation is a compulsory part of a portfolio section with specific learning outcomes, a pre-printed document may already be available – check with your personal tutor if this is the case.

As part of your learning journey, you may decide to spend a day observing or working with a health professional in another area of practice to gain insight into his or her role and expertise. This would inform your knowledge of the area of care chosen and may help to improve your practice further through transfer of skills and knowledge learnt from the day.

It is useful to set yourself objectives for the day and have a clear idea of the outcomes you want to achieve. Again it is useful to discuss this with the health professional and your mentor prior to the visit to ensure that the outcomes and objectives are achievable in the time allocated.

A pre-prepared witness statement/testimonial form is useful to take along, again to ensure the areas you have highlighted are addressed. This also gives relevant healthcare professionals guidance in what you hope to achieve from the time spent with them, and is also a means of verifying the time allocated.

From these visits and observations, it would be beneficial to write a reflection to accompany the witness statements. This would demonstrate your understanding of the knowledge and skills gained, and how you hope to take this forward in improving practice. It would also give an opportunity to formulate an action plan to structure your next steps in applying the learning from this area.

Testimonials are similar to witness statements and can be utilised as evidence within your portfolio to support how you are currently working and learning in practice. These are mainly narrative and express the writer's opinions and views on your professional practice, progress, strengths and areas for improvement.

A request for a testimonial may be made to your mentor, placement leader, personal tutor, a colleague, or other health professional with whom you have spent a period of time.

A pre-printed form is not usually applicable in this instance, although you may want to negotiate areas for comments with the writer beforehand and justify how this will improve your learning. *Figure 3.6* is an example of a format that could be used. Again, a piece of reflective writing could accompany the testimonial to promote learning.

It is generally accepted that if people agree to write a witness statement or testimonial, that it will be seen by others such as the student's tutor, supervisor, etc. However, it is important that you inform all signatories of the purpose of their statements, that their comments will be included within your portfolio and who this will be viewed by.

It is good practice to include a list of the names of the people who have

Testimonial for: ....

Date: ....

Length of time worked with student: ....

Areas for consideration: ....

....

....

....

Strengths: ....

....

....

....

Areas for improvement: ....

....

....

....

Attitude, skills, knowledge: ....

....

....

....

Signature and designation ....

Figure 3.6. Example of a testimonial form.

written and signed documents within your portfolio, with their signed agreement for their inclusion.

It is imperative that while reflecting on critical incidents, case studies and situations occurring within practice, that names of patients, colleagues, and placements are given pseudonyms to protect confidentiality. This should be declared within the introduction of your portfolio. Care must be taken when including emails where the message is intended for the recipient only. This also includes group emails where other email addresses may be visible. Always check with your mentor, supervisor or award leader in relation to specific confidentiality issues necessary within your field of practice and adhere to Nursing and Midwifery Council guidelines (2002).

Minutes of meetings, mentor discussions and clinical supervision

Meetings you attend as part of your learning journey can be interesting and inspiring. They can also give you a greater understanding of a certain organisation, network, policy, service or situation. As you gain confidence, they may be a useful forum to voice your opinions on the issues under discussion.

You may wish to include the following minutes of meetings:

* ward/general practice meetings
* team/staff meetings
* student representative meetings
* academic/curriculum development meetings
* health authority meetings
* board meetings, ie. clinical governance, commissioning, continuing professional development, etc.
* specialist service meetings, ie. diabetes, public health, screening, discharge planning, etc.
* action learning sets.

Attendees of meetings included must be contacted for their permission for inclusion. Unless this is obtained, their names must be deleted from the document that is submitted within the portfolio.

Mentor discussions can also be included as evidence of learning and can be useful to show progression over a period of time. These may be in narrative form to support other methods of evidence such as witness statements or observations of clinical skills to assess competence, or they may be as a reflection of the discussions you have had concerning a particular situation or case. Again, always adhere to the issued criteria and learning outcomes of your portfolio to ascertain the academic level of evidence needed if relevant.

Details of clinical supervision meetings may also be recorded within your portfolio. It can be that, when you have thought about a certain situation and have formed opinions, on discussing it with colleagues and peers you realise that there is more than one way of looking at the circumstances involved. By analysing the components, and having other opinions or views that could add to your knowledge base, may make you aware of issues of which you might not previously have thought. Again, the level of detail for the writing of these meetings will depend on the structure and criteria of evidence required. It may be a good idea to utilise a reflective module to give more depth and analysis if needed.

Presentations

A useful way of providing evidence of learning is through a presentation. This can be to fellow students, colleagues, patient forums, healthcare organisations, including voluntary agencies and charities, practice teams, and health forums, groups and associations. Presentations can also be useful on an individual one-to-one basis to demonstrate learning, progression and understanding. Presentations may be to your mentor/supervisor, personal tutor, or manager.

Whichever format you feel is most appropriate, a presentation can be used to demonstrate competence of your skills and knowledge gained, disseminate the learning that has taken place through analysis of the subject area, and identify recommendations for future learning and formulation of action plans. Therefore an effective understanding of presentation skills is required.

Ways of including a presentation within your portfolio could be through:

* copies of slides used in presentations (with notes, session plans, etc.)
* witness statements from observers/mentors
* evaluations from audiences and mentors
* reflection
* videos of presentations.

Many nurses find speaking at a conference, small meeting or to a group of colleagues daunting. However, as nurses develop a political voice for both the patient and the profession, it is important that they acquire effective presentation skills in order to communicate their message in a way that results in a change in understanding or opinion (Hadfield-Law, 2001). Whether it is a presentation to a patient or to conference delegates, nursing professionals have a responsibility to share and disseminate knowledge.

Preparing effectively is the key to a successful presentation. The most important areas to consider when planning a presentation include:

■ *Who is the audience?* Health professionals, students, patients, managers etc.? Is the group large or small, do they know you? Will the academic level or expertise of the audience be known, eg. a presentation required as part of an undergraduate assessment to academics may be very different from a presentation giving information to managers to secure resources.

- *What is the purpose of the presentation?* Is it a seminar format, to promote discussion and debate to gain opinion, to give information, to persuade, ie. bidding for resources, requirement of an interview process, as part of a summative academic assessment. What do you want the audience to know, think, feel or do when they leave the presentation?
- *What are the aims/objectives?* Be clear about what you want to present. An overall aim followed by specific objectives may be useful in setting direction and giving structure. However, if the presentation involves stimulating debate, a broader aim may be sufficient. When forming part of an academic assessment, the related learning outcomes should be adhered to.
- *What is the time frame?* Always check and confirm this, it is necessary that your presentation remains within the time allocated. Focus on your key points, do not try to include everything you know about the subject area. Clarify to the audience when you are prepared to take questions, ie. throughout or at the close of your presentation. This will need to be included within the time frame.

Making a start

An interesting or unusual start to the presentation will capture the interest of the audience, as will an obvious enthusiasm from the speaker. Therefore, know your subject area well. This will help you feel more confident and reduce anxiety. Instead of saying,

My presentation today is about health promotion and these are the aims and objectives of the session. These are some definitions of health ...

Why not try,

What does being healthy mean to you? [Thought shower asking members of the audience to share their views]

This suggests that just within this group, everyone has a different view on what 'being healthy' means. You could then continue,

Let us see how these compare with some definitions of health

Instead of saying,

My presentation today is about coronary heart disease and how to reduce modifiable risk factors. These are the main risk factors ... This is the current evidence that suggests ways of how we can reduce these risks...

Why not try:

My presentation today concerns the management of coronary heart disease. What do we currently know? Here's a quick quiz to get you thinking. Displayed are a few statements which could be true or false... [list these on slides and ask the audience to raise their hands if they think they are true or false, or use the format of a quiz show, etc.]

Anecdotal cases from practice can be used to good effect in bringing the subject to life – this may be through humour, sadness, even horror. Again, remember to ensure anonymity. An interesting case study, delivered articulately can make a great start to a presentation, which then sets the scene for the subject area and can link to the main points for discussion.

An obvious way of capturing interest is through audiovisual aids which will be discussed in more detail later. A video clip or relevant images related to your subject area can bring a presentation to life if used effectively.

Reducing anxiety

Practise, practise and practise again. If you are well prepared and know the presentation thoroughly, you will feel more confident and less anxious. Present to family members, friends, colleagues and ask for their constructive feedback. Ensure you arrive in plenty of time for the presentation to arrange the environment and seating if necessary, check resources, and to meet members of the audience as appropriate. If you are anxious, your mouth will become dry so ensure you have a drink on hand. Always smile, you cannot look worried or frown and smile at the same time.

It is useful to remember reaction to fear can be positive. Adrenalin that is produced by fear can stimulate creative energy and enthusiasm and can actually enhance your presentation delivery (Davidhizar and Dowd, 1997).

Delivery

Structure your presentation to its purpose and the audience involved, identifying key points and using extra material if time allows. Do not read notes from sheets of paper as it can be distracting and surprisingly noisy. If you must read prepared notes, it is better to use small numbered cards. However if you are fully prepared this may not be needed.

Speak in a clear voice that can be heard by all, and try to vary the pitch, tone and pace of your voice throughout. Maintain eye contact with your audience, and do not stand still in one place throughout the presentation if this is appropriate. Involve the audience if possible. Show enthusiasm, the impact of non-verbal aspects of communication such as dress, body language, tone and facial expression are said to be at least 93% of the message that is actually received (Weissman, 2003).

Visual aids

Audiovisual aids can enhance a presentation, but ensure you are familiar with these methods prior to delivery and take time to practise. It is a good idea to have a back-up plan if technology fails, ie. back-up disc, acetates, poster.

If using a power point presentation, ensure slides are not overloaded with information. This can detract from the points you are trying to make. Whichever audiovisual aids you choose, they must be clear and visible to the whole audience. Care should be taken when choosing background and font colours, as they can look quite different when portrayed on a large screen.

Concluding

It is important to summarise the key points of your presentation, and you may want to re-visit the original aims. Again, as at the start of the presentation, ensure the conclusion ends on an interesting, poignant, humorous note which the audience will remember. Practise your concluding remarks until you feel confident you are word perfect and do not need to read from notes. This will be your last chance to get your point across, so make it count.

You may want to conclude by asking the audience a question, making a controversial statement to stimulate debate, asking what the audience have learned from the presentation, if it is a teaching session, and how they will apply this learning to their practice, or by requesting and taking questions from the audience.

Being able to articulate effectively, whether to small or large groups, can be an extremely effective skill in facilitating your career advancement within the nursing profession.

Summary

There is a wide variety of evidence that can be used to support achievement of learning and competence within your portfolio. Always ensure that the requirements are understood, and take time to clarify any points that appear unclear. For example, is a word limit stated, is there a minimum and/or maximum number of reflections needed, will a CD Rom/video be acceptable as part of the evidence submitted?

Ascertain if there is availability for a colleague, tutor, manager or mentor to review the portfolio at regular intervals (if appropriate or relevant) to give constructive feedback and identify areas for improvement.

It is important that you plan and prepare effectively to ensure that the evidence included is relevant to what is required.

References

Atkins S, Murphy K (1994) Reflective practice. *Nursing Standard* **8**(39): 49–54

Borton T (1970) *Reach, Touch and Teach*. McGraw-Hill, London

Carper B (1978) Fundamental patterns of knowing in nursing. *Advances in Nursing Science* **1**(10): 13–23

Covey SR (1989) *The Habits of Highly Effective People: Lessons in Personal Change*. Simon and Schuster, London

Cranton P (1994) *Understanding and Promoting Transfomative Learning*. Jossey-Bass, San Francisco

Davidhizar R, Dowd S (1997) The art of giving an effective presentation. *Health Care Supervisor* **15**(3): 25–32

Dewey J (1938) *Experience and Education*. Macmillan, New York

Gibbs G (1988) *Learning by Doing: A Guide to Teaching and Learning Methods*. Further Education Unit, Oxford Polytechnic, Oxford

Hadfield-Law L (2001) Presentation skills for nurses: How to prepare more effectively. *Br J Nursing* **10**(18): 1208–12

Hannigan B (2001) A discussion of the strengths and weaknesses of 'reflection' in nursing practice and education. *J Clin Nursing* **10**(2): 278–83

Jarvis P (1992) Reflective practice in nursing. *Nurse Education Today* **12**: 174–81

Johns C (2000) *Becoming a Reflective Practitioner*. Blackwell Publishing, Oxford

Kolb D (1984) *Experiential Learning: Experience as the source of Learning and Development*. Prentice Hall, New York

Mezirow J (1998) On critical reflection. *Adult Ed Quarterly* **45**: 185–98

Nursing and Midwifery Council (2002) *The PREP Handbook*. NMC, London

Rolfe G, Freshwater D, Jasper M (2001) *Critical Reflection for Nursing and the Helping Professions: A User's Guide*. Palgrave MacMillan, Hampshire

Saylor C (1990) Reflection and professional education: Art, science and competency. *Nurse Educator* **15**: 8–11

Schon D (1987) *The Reflective Practitioner*. Jossey-Bass, San Francisco

Teekman B (2000) Exploring reflective thinking in nursing practice. *J Adv Nursing* **31**: 1125–35

Van Manen M (1991) *The Tact of Teaching*. NY State University Press, New York

Weissman J (2003) *Presenting to Win: The Art of Telling Your Story*. Prentice Hall, New Jersey

CHAPTER 4

Organising your portfolio logically and effectively

Kay Norman

Introduction

Whatever the purpose of compiling a portfolio, whether it is as part of an academic assessment, evidence to present at interview, or as part of a continuing professional development profile, it is imperative that it is organised effectively. The amount of evidence produced, the format, and the indexing may differ depending on its use but it must be logical and easy to navigate.

This chapter discusses ways in which a portfolio may be organised, including examples of index systems, cross-referencing, and format styles that could be used. It also considers curriculum vitae as a useful component within a portfolio.

Organisational systems

The main focus when organising a portfolio is to ensure that the material included corresponds to the requirements. For example, as part of an academic assessment, evidence is required to show achievement of a learning outcome.

To support an interview process, evidence of continual professional development and contents pertinent to the role applied for is needed, such as educational certificates, courses attended, testimonials, etc.

As part of a pre-registration nursing programme, certain requirements may be necessary and a predetermined structure may be advised. It may be necessary to organise evidence into 'years of study', 'module sections' or 'key skills'. Key skills are discussed in more detail in *Chapter 5*.

It is important that the evidence provided shows learning and progression and includes all necessary documentation.

A checklist is often helpful as a reminder of what is needed:

- *Presentation folder*: this should be sturdy and large enough for evidence to be inserted and located easily. Double ring binder folders with a secure fastening are most appropriate.

- Contents page: use a font in 12pt size with bold, italic or underlining formatting as appropriate.
- Evidence should be clear and concise and typed in a plain font. Use the same font, style and format throughout if possible.
- Evidence and inserts should be placed in clear plastic wallets to prevent fraying unless directed otherwise.
- Check that all required evidence and documentation is included.
- Use sections to organise evidence logically as required.
- Use plastic section dividers (card can become shabby).
- Use a clear, logical index system which is introduced and explained.
- Use a cross-referencing system and ensure it is introduced and easily understood.
- Include introductory, conclusion and summary sections.
- Include an introductory statement for each section if this is appropriate.
- Include biographical details if required.
- Ensure confidentiality statements are included and that anonymity is maintained.
- Add an appendices section as necessary.

Index systems

A clear logical indexing system should direct the reader to all the evidence submitted within the portfolio. You will know your portfolio and its contents well, and may feel confident that the evidence can easily be located. However it is important that you also take advice from colleagues with regard to the organisation and format. It may be that someone else cannot locate evidence due to an inadequate or complex indexing system. Therefore enlist the help of others to read, review and locate evidence within your portfolio to highlight areas for improvement. A peer group may be useful, where members can review each others' portfolios and give comments. This is also an opportunity to share ideas with others relating to indexing systems and organisation of portfolios.

Whichever system you decide to use, make sure you are comfortable with it. Despite your colleague's organisational system looking perfect, if you find it difficult to understand and apply, do not use it. Often the simplest index systems are the best and easiest to navigate. Whichever system you decide to use, ensure that it is clear and logical, and demonstrated within the contents page.

Use the same system throughout the portfolio to avoid confusion. Examples of index systems include:

- Labelled sections relating to requirements/learning outcomes, where each

---

Contents

Figure 4.1. Example of a portfolio contents page.

section has one learning outcome and all the related evidence for that particular outcome.
- Labelled sections according to the types of evidence included. For example, a section related to reflections, a section related to witness statements, a section related to SLOT analyses.
- Clearly typed page numbers.
- Coloured inserts/labels which could include self-adhesive coloured dots which can be located on the upper right hand corner of the evidence included. Be aware that these can become unstuck, so ensure they are secure.
- Labelled alphabetical sections and inserts.
- Grids and/or diagrams that direct the reader to appropriate evidence.

You may want to organise your portfolio in sections relating to learning outcomes. *Figure 4.1* gives an example of a contents page within a portfolio.

Figure 4.2 gives an example of an extract from an introduction section relating to an academic assessed portfolio. Be mindful to adhere to specific word count requirements, which may influence the length of your introduction section. Ensure the introduction 'sets the scene' for the reader and clearly indicates what has been achieved and how this will be demonstrated within the portfolio.

Figure 4.3 is an extract from a section within the portfolio where cross-referencing is highlighted. Page numbers are used to clearly indicate which other sections provide evidence of achievement for this outcome through cross-referencing. You could also use different colours for different sections.

Introduction

On commencement of this module, I had already accumulated some knowledge within this area and had three years' previous experience in mentoring students in higher education. However, throughout the three terms spent studying this area, I have gained invaluable knowledge and understanding of learning theories, wider experience of teaching and learning strategies, and improved skills in critical reflection in order to inform and improve my teaching role.

I have also gained a deeper understanding of my strengths and limitations within this role, and acknowledging how others' perceptions can help in my self-awareness, ultimately leading to increased critical reflective skills and role performance.

Throughout my studies, I have questioned my own and the organisation's strategies of teaching and learning, tried to build on new strategies learned, and tried to disseminate this increased knowledge as appropriate; not only through my role as lecturer, but also through a conference presentation and publishing an article within a peer reviewed journal to reach a wider audience.

The contents of this portfolio portray an enjoyable and rewarding journey of learning, inherent to which includes evidence relating to the achievement of the required learning outcomes. Throughout this learning journey, a philosophy that has been instrumental in changing my perspective on teaching and learning is portrayed by Tyler (1949): 'Learning takes place through the active behaviour of the student, it is what he does that he learns, not what the teacher does.'

Therefore I realise that my fundamental task is to encourage and ensure students engage in learning activities that will contribute to them achieving the learning required and hopefully beyond. I see my role as teaching students how to learn, by developing independent inquiry, not just what to learn by giving information.

On reflecting on my practice role, I had always endeavoured to help and support students achieve their goals which would ultimately led to success. However, I now recognise that in giving this intensive support, it may have been me directing the student rather than allowing students to direct their learning and developing their own learning strategies in order to achieve their outcomes.

From this theme, I have also reflected on assessment and how as mentors we may want to control this process, with many students concentrating only on this component of the module/course when centralising their learning efforts (Jarvis *et al*, 2004). Through critical reflection I have tried to develop other ways of assessing, relating to practical and theoretical components of programmes I am currently involved with. This has included peer and student self-assessment, work-based learning, and assessed learning outcomes in practice by CPTs and mentors.

Included within this portfolio are critical reflections of observed teaching sessions, along with reflections of the teaching practice and activities necessary within this module. Witness statements and testimonials from managers, colleagues and students support these in justifying achievement of the required learning outcomes.

Some names have been deleted to protect confidentiality, although by the very nature of witness statements/testimonials, they remain in their original format.

Figure 4.2. An example of a general introduction section within an assessed portfolio.

Introduction

On self-assessing my communication and working relationships with students and other mentors, I felt that this was a personal strength in many ways, but also appreciated that there is always room for improvement. As a mentor myself, I can also reflect and see through their 'lens', and their role and potential concerns in this area when developing appropriate supportive relationships, leading to a greater understanding of how students integrate into a new practice setting and assisting with this process (Brookfield, 1995). Consequently, I also reflected on my previous experience as a specialist practice student to give some insight into how students may be supported.

Throughout this course, I have learned much about communication with students, mentors and colleagues. Although it can be said that communication is the essence of nursing (Hogston and Simpson, 1999), the skills required within an educational role in this area can be varied including individual and group interactions, which, through reflection, can be continually improved upon. From my initial 360° feedback, I have reflected on how others' perceptions can be at odds with one's own perceptions. Following this I have continued to develop supportive strategies within my role involving students and mentors, and now feel able to give this support without necessarily adopting a 'parenting' and directing role. This allows the student and mentor the opportunity to lead the discussions and reflect on their own learning needs and how I can help to facilitate these (Jarvis *et al*, 2004).

I have gained further knowledge of approaches that could be adopted through the observation of my teaching practice and tutorials, and subsequent discussions with my supervisor. This has encouraged me to reflect on my own personal style of communication within my role, and accept that alternative methods of communication may be necessary at different times and within varying situations (Quinn, 2000).

Evidence relating to the achievement of this outcome is supplied in
Section 4	*pp 7–14*

Further evidence is supplied in
Section 4	*pp 4, 6*
Section 5	*pp 14–20*
Section 6	*pp 21–22*
Section 8	*p 40*

Figure 4.3. Example of a section introduction in a portfolio with cross-referencing.

Learning outcome	Year 1	Year 2	Year 3
To evaluate critically and demonstrate understanding of concepts pertinent to healthcare	Reflection on collaborative working: **See Section A Insert 3** Minutes of multidisciplinary meeting within practice **See Section B Insert 5** Discussion with mentor regarding breaking down barriers of traditional nursing roles **See Section C Insert 10**	Minutes from patient forum **See Section B Insert 6** Reflection on patient participation within a hospital environment **See Section A Insert 4** Testimonial from ward manager **See Section D Insert 1**	Concept analysis on leadership **See Section E Insert 2** Reflection on managing a nursing bay within a medical unit under supervision **See Section A Insert 6** Testimonial from team leader **See Section D Insert 4** SLOT analysis **See Section F Insert 3**
	Signature of mentor/CPT/ supervisor:	*Signature of mentor/CPT/ supervisor:*	*Signature of mentor/CPT/ supervisor:*

Figure 4.4. Cross-referencing table.

Figure 4.4 is an example of a table that can be used to locate and cross-reference evidence of achievement relating to a specific learning outcome. Alphabetically labelled, coloured divider sections and numbered inserts within the portfolio will provide easy access and direction to the relevant documentation.

Curriculum vitae

In some circumstances, for example within pre-registration nursing programmes, it may be beneficial to include a curriculum vitae (CV) within the introduction of the portfolio.

This presents clearly your biographical details, educational and employment background, and gives an opportunity to present 'a picture' of yourself to the reader. There are many formats for writing a CV, which are generally accessible from libraries and internet sources. However, it is important that the CV is meaningful to you, appropriate for its specific use, and is well presented. A CV can be described as a marketing tool to sell your achievements.

Areas to consider when compiling a CV:

- Avoid lengthy descriptions, bullet points are clearer and stand out to the reader.
- Ensure a clear, simple font (eg. Aerial 12pt) on good quality white paper.
- Arrange data clearly, logically and simply in chronological order.
- Always check for spelling and grammatical errors.

A CV should include:

- Name.
- Address.
- Telephone/email contact.
- Employment history.
- Skills summary: main skills you can demonstrate. Use key words, not lengthy descriptions.
- Educational summary: again only list what is relevant and recent. Within this section you may want to include short courses, study days, etc. or you may want to list these under a separate heading – 'additional study'.
- Objectives/goals: this gives you the opportunity to demonstrate your ambitions and goals for your future career, but ensure they are realistic. Again, a short concise statement that informs what your short- and long-term aspirations are, and the type of position that you are looking for is all that is needed. Long descriptions may not be read.
- Achievements: these could include personal and professional attainments,

such as awards, overcoming barriers to achieve a personal or professional goal, outstanding academic results, leading a project, nomination for a caring/nursing prize, etc. This may help to inform the reader of your determination, hard work and leadership skills and give a further insight into your characteristics. Again, keep these achievements recent and relevant.

■ Activities/hobbies: provide a short statement detailing any activities or hobbies you are involved with. This may include voluntary work, sports activities, etc.

A CV should be updated regularly, as and when changes occur. A CV required for an employment interview may need amending depending on the post you are applying for. For example, you may be required to supply additional information on why you have applied for the post, why you feel you are suitable for the role, etc. In these circumstances you may want to 'tailor' your CV to encompass skills related to the job description and desirable criteria stated for the position.

Summary

The effective organisation of a portfolio is essential to ensure its purpose is fulfilled. Clear, logical signposting to relevant information within the portfolio should be discussed with colleagues and supervisors who can also give you ideas for any improvements that could be made to the structure and format.

Take pride in, and enjoy this component of portfolio development. You should feel a real sense of achievement on completion of a well-organised and clearly presented portfolio.

References

Brookfield SD (1995) *Becoming a Critically Reflective Teacher*. Jossey Bass, San Francisco

Hogston R, Simpson PM (1999) *Foundations of Nursing Practice*. MacMillan, Basingstoke

Jarvis P, Holford J, Griffin C (2004) *The Theory and Practice of Learning* (2nd edn) Routledge Falmer, London

Tyler RW (1949) *Basic Principles of Curriculum and Instruction*. Chicago University Press, Chicago

Quinn FM (2000) *Principles and Practice of Nurse Education* (4th edn) Nelson Thornes, London

CHAPTER 5

Use of key skills in portfolios to enhance employability

Nicky Genders

Introduction

This chapter discusses the use of key skills as a framework for portfolio development. It also focuses on the use of key skills to enhance employability. There are many ways to organise a portfolio and the use of key skills is one which has been adopted in some areas. The organisation of the portfolio and its evidence is discussed in *Chapter 3*, and as the portfolio exists in many forms this has also been discussed within other chapters in this book.

The focus of this chapter is on the development of key skills within the portfolio. All portfolios will include evidence of your key skill development but not all portfolios will acknowledge key skills explicitly.

There are six key skill areas discussed here: communication, application of number, information technology, working with others, improving own learning and problem solving.

If we take the example of improving own learning and performance as a key skill, the development of a portfolio that includes reflection and self-assessment will inherently develop this key skill and in turn the development of the portfolio provides evidence for the skill. But we need to be aware of what we are developing our portfolio for – is its primary purpose to demonstrate nursing competence or to demonstrate key skills? The majority of portfolios in nurse education use models which serve to demonstrate nursing competence against specific standards or criteria. A portfolio may also begin using one model and then evolve into something quite different. For example, a portfolio may be an integrated model demonstrating a range of competence gained across a pre-registration nursing course. This portfolio may then be adapted at the point of employment to demonstrate specific role competence or to demonstrate the key skills gained throughout the nursing programme.

There are many portfolio models in use in nursing and nurse education, therefore this chapter focuses on the broad aspects of key skill development within the portfolio.

Table 5.1. Qualifications and Curriculum Authority key skills

---

Communication
- Oral communication
- Written communication
- Reading

Application of number
- Interpreting information
- Carrying out calculations
- Interpreting results and presenting findings

Information technology
- Finding and selecting information
- Developing information
- Presenting information

Problem solving
- Identifying problems
- Considering solutions
- Reviewing and evaluating outcomes

Working with others
- Planning the work
- Working to identified objectives
- Reviewing progress

Improving own learning and performance

What are key skills?

Although the term key skills is much used and can encompass many aspects of skill development, in the context of this chapter, key skills are those skills described by the Qualifications and Curriculum Authority (2004) as highlighted in *Table 5.1*.

Key skills have been described as those skills which are useful in education, training, work and life generally (Qualifications and Curriculum Authority, 2004). These skills have been built into a qualification framework used within schools, colleges and higher education. Over 300 000 key skill qualifications were awarded in 2003/2004 in the UK with the majority of centres being further education colleges or private training providers (Department for Education and Skills, 1995). Each of the key skills includes a specification and they are assessable at five levels. These assessments lead to specific key skill qualifications and some people putting together a portfolio may already have gained key skill qualifications at school or college. Although very few higher education institutions offer key skills qualifications many have mapped key skills against the curriculum and you

---

Table. 5.2. Qualifications and Curriculum Authority Specification: Communication level 2

Evidence must show you can

Take part in a group discussion
- Make clear and relevant contribution in a way that suits your purpose and situation
- Respond appropriately to others
- Help to move the discussion forward

Give a talk of at least four minutes
- Speak clearly in a way that suits your subject, purpose and situation
- Keep to the subject and structure your talk to help listeners follow what you are saying
- Use appropriate ways to support your main points

Read and summarise information from at least two documents about the same subject. Each document must be a minimum of 500 words long
- Select and read relevant documents
- Identify accurately the main points, ideas and lines of reasoning
- Summarise the information to suit your purpose

Write two different types of documents each one giving different information. One document must be at least 50 words long
- Present relevant information in a format that suits the purpose
- Use a structure and style of writing to suit your purpose
- Spell, punctuate and use grammar accurately
- Make your meaning clear

Use at least one image either to obtain information or to convey information in your discussion, your talk or one of the documents you write in order to help the audience/reader understand the points you are making.

---

may find that there is specific guidance on the achievement of key skills if you are undertaking a module, course or programme.

For assessment purposes key skills are identified then broken down further into competence statements, against which assessment may take place (Qualifications and Curriculum Authority, 2004). For example the competence statement for communication at level 2 is shown in *Table 5.2* and for level 4 in *Table 5.3*.

These examples illustrate the differences in key skill levels and the requirements you would have to meet if you were undertaking formal key skill qualifications. The specifications for all key skills can be found at www.qca.

Table 5.3. Qualifications and Curriculum Authority specification: Communication level 4

Evidence must show you can

Develop a strategy for using communication skills over an extended period of time
- Clearly identify the outcomes you hope to achieve
- Plan your use of communication skills, and make a reasoned selection of methods for achieving the quality of outcomes required
- Identify relevant sources and research the information

Monitor progress and adapt your strategy as necessary to achieve the quality of outcomes required in work involving at least one group discussion and one document of 1000 words or more about a complex subject
- Evaluate and synthesise information from different sources
- Communicate relevant information accurately and effectively using a form, structure and style that suits your purpose, and respond perceptively to contributions from others
- Monitor and critically reflect on your use of communication skills, adapting your strategy as necessary to produce the quality of outcomes required

Evaluate your overall strategy and present the outcomes from you work, using at least one formal oral presentation, include a variety of verbal, visual and other techniques to illustrate your points
- Organise and present clearly relevant information, illustrating what you say in ways that suit the purpose, subject and audience
- Vary use of vocabulary and grammatical expression to convey particular effects, enable fine distinctions to be made, achieve emphasis and engage the audience
- Assess the effectiveness of your strategy, including factors that had an impact on the outcomes, and identify ways of further developing your communication skills

---

org.uk. Using these examples of key skill specifications it can be seen that while undertaking many pre- and post-registration nursing courses key skills are being developed.

If you have undertaken key skill qualifications at school or college you may have a clear understanding of the different areas of key skill development that relate to nursing competence. While it is not suggested that all nurses undertake formal key skill qualifications if we use the broad headings of the key skills we can see that a portfolio can be focused, should we chose to, around these transferable skills.

Nursing encompasses all six key skills. However, it cannot be assumed that all nurses automatically possess these skills and therefore the curriculum both in pre-registration and post-registration education develops them as essential, transferable skills. Historically, nurses have been seen to be less confident in some of the skills, in particular information technology and application of number (numeracy). Lack of this latter key skill has caused drug dosage calculation errors, and nurses' abilities to calculate drugs effectively have been brought into question (Jukes and Gilchrist, 2006). This has led to changes to many nursing curricula to include calculation/numeracy testing where this was previously absent and for some admissions departments to acknowledge key skill qualifications in numeracy at level two or above as evidence of numerical skill. This is a very specific example of the link between nursing practice and key skill development and the way in which this has been addressed at an educational level. For many of the other key skills their links are embedded into the curriculum.

Even where the key skills are not as explicit, in many courses or programmes of study key skills are often developed further, for example:

- *Nurse prescribing course*: focuses specifically on the development of application of number for drug calculations.
- *Nursing leadership module*: focuses specifically on the development of 'working with others'.
- *Research module*: focuses specifically on the development of information technology and problem solving skills.

A further example of how nursing specifically develops the key skills can be seen when we compare the Nursing and Midwifery Council standards of proficiency for pre-registration nursing to the key skill areas. *Table 5.4* shows how the key skills set out in *Table 5.1* are evident within all pre-registration nursing curricula. They are not always explicitly assessed and you may not have focused on these skills when developing your portfolio but there will be evidence of the development of these skills.

Evidence of key skills within the portfolio

There are many forms of portfolio as previously discussed and evidence of key skill development may be subtle and implicit rather than explicit. If you have developed or are developing a portfolio you may wish to make the key skills more explicit or you may even decide to develop your own key skills portfolio. For example, a key skills portfolio could be appropriate preparation for a job interview as it focuses your evidence on those transferable skills. The following examples show the types of evidence that may be used in a key skills portfolio.

Table 5.4. Nursing and Midwifery Council (2004) standards of proficiency which can be compared to the key skills in Table 5.1

- Manage oneself, one's practice and that of others in accordance with the NMC Code of Professional Conduct: standards for conduct, performance and ethics (the Code) recognising one's own abilities and limitations
- Practise in accordance with an ethical and legal framework which ensures the primacy of patient and client interest and well-being and respects confidentiality
- Practise in a fair and anti-discriminatory way, acknowledging the differences in beliefs and cultural practices of individuals or groups
- Engage in, develop and disengage from therapeutic relationships through the use of appropriate communication and interpersonal skills
- Create and utilise opportunities to promote the health and well-being of patients, clients and groups
- Undertake and document a comprehensive, systematic and accurate nursing assessment of the physical, psychological, social and spiritual needs of patients, clients and communities.
- Formulate and document a plan of nursing care, where possible in partnership with patients, clients, their carers and family friends, within a framework of informed consent
- Based on the best available evidence, apply knowledge and an appropriate repertoire of skills indicative of safe nursing practice
- Provide a rationale for the nursing care delivered which takes account of social, cultural, spiritual, legal, political and economic influences
- Evaluate and document the outcomes of nursing and other interventions
- Demonstrate sound clinical judgement across a range of differing professional and care delivery contexts
- Contribute to public protection by creating and maintaining a safe environment of care through the use of quality assurance and risk management strategies
- Demonstrate knowledge of effective inter-professional working practices which respect and utilise the contributions of members of the health and social care team
- Delegate duties to others, as appropriate, ensuring that they are supervised and monitored
- Demonstrate key skills
- Demonstrate a commitment to the need for CPD and personal supervision activities in order to enhance knowledge, skills, values and attitudes needed for safe and effective nursing practice
- Enhance the professional development and safe practice of others through peer support, leadership, supervision and teaching

Communication

A range of communication skills may be demonstrated in a nursing context including verbal and non-verbal skills and written forms of communication. Patient records, day-to-day communication, notes from ward meetings and multi-disciplinary team meetings are all examples of the frequent use of a range of communications skills. There may also be specific incidents where you have used your communications skills in a non-routine way, for example, supporting a relative following bereavement or presenting a training session for staff. Higher level skills may include developing a communication strategy within a specific role. These 'critical incidents' may be reflected upon within your portfolio and used as examples of key skill development.

Evidence of verbal and written communication skills may include practice reports, posters and feedback from assignments identifying good written communication. You may have examples of seminar presentations or similar and annotated bibliographies can highlight your reading. You may have included an appraisal report that highlights skills in developing a communication strategy.

Application of number

As previously noted the application of number or numeracy within nursing has been the focus of criticism within the literature. Being able to demonstrate numeracy is becoming increasingly important in the nursing context and a portfolio that clearly highlights your skills will enhance your employability.

This may include evidence from drug calculation simulations in clinical practice and classroom-based tests. Assignments which include statistical analysis could also be included.

Information technology

Information technology within healthcare is developing rapidly from ward-based new technologies for direct patient care to computerised integrated health records. The use of these technologies alongside skills in data handling, word processing and the management of statistics is becoming crucial within the healthcare arena. This may include evidence from assignments, practice including use of computer-based records, and the use of classroom technology such as Blackboard and WebCT.

Improving own learning, working with others and problem solving

Improving your own learning is a key skill underpinning portfolio development and a career within health care. The process of identifying your learning needs and action planning to meet these needs creates the opportunity to improve your learning. Lifelong learning has been a key concept for some time within healthcare with the Department of Health in 2001 producing its report *Working Together – Learning Together: A Framework for Life Long Learning in the NHS*. This report argues strongly that lifelong learning improves patient care. In a changing workforce employers expect healthcare workers to be able to identify their strengths and weaknesses and identify their learning needs (Hull *et al*, 2005). The appraisal system and other performance management techniques support this approach encouraging self-assessment and personal development planning. Much of the literature acknowledges a shift in thinking in training and education over the last two decades as learning becomes more learner centred and the healthcare workforce becomes more flexible and dynamic (Hull *et al*, 2005). The portfolio puts learners at the centre of their learning and at its best the portfolio becomes a vehicle for dynamic learning.

Being able to work with others is a further crucial skill within the nursing context. Healthcare workers work in single and multi-disciplinary teams in order to deliver effective patient care. Understanding professional boundaries and the culture of the various professional groups can ensure appropriate working relationships.

Complex problem solving is an inherent part of the nursing role. Schon (1983) wrote extensively about reflective practice and the professional noting that a number of issues emerged when looking at the tasks and roles professional groups take on. It was noted that the problems faced on a day-to-day basis required complex problem solving skills and that decision making was based on a detailed knowledge base. The use of this knowledge base and the related skills was also seen as contextual and that professional knowledge is more than a set of expert skills. Benner's work is also noteworthy here in acknowledging the changing nature of problem solving approaches as the nurse moves from 'novice' to 'expert' (Benner, 1984). The observations of these writers, and many more, confirm the importance of this key skill in nursing. Evidence for these three key skills can come from a wide range of sources, eg. practice reports, simulations and assignments. You may have reports from specific multi-disciplinary placements or reflections. The process of 'action planning' within the portfolio contributes to the development of 'improving own learning' as discussed in previous chapters.

Self-assessment and key skills

Identifying evidence, reviewing that evidence and selecting it for inclusion into the portfolio requires skills of self-assessment. Self-assessment gives you ownership of your evidence and therefore your portfolio. However, choosing evidence from a wide range of sources to meet the needs of your portfolio development is a skill that should be developed. You need to know who you are developing your portfolio for and what its ultimate aim is. Do you have control over its content or is there a more rigid structure? Once you are clear on these questions and, for the purposes of this chapter, assuming you would like to build a key skills focused portfolio we can use a process of self-assessment:

- Review the key skills that the portfolio hopes to demonstrate (this may include levels of achievement).
- Identify evidence that meets specific key skills achievement.
- Examine that evidence with the following questions in mind:
  - Is this the best piece of evidence I have to demonstrate competence in this key skill area?
  - How much of the key skill does it cover and do I need further evidence to support this?
  - Does it reflect my knowledge and skills?
  - Does it present me in the best possible way?
- There are also some basic questions to ask which apply to all types of evidence in portfolios:
  - Is it relevant ?
  - Is it valid?
  - Is it authentic?

The following is an example of self-assessment.

Annie has arranged to see her mentor to review her portfolio and would like to discuss the key skills evidence she has included.

Annie has recently received the results of her drug calculation assessment and was pleased with such a high grade. She feels though that this test alone does not fully demonstrate her competence so has decided also to present her last placement report. Prior to this placement Annie had put together an action plan to develop her drug calculation skills in the clinical setting. Her placement mentor supported this and allowed Annie every opportunity for supervised practice in this area. The placement used a range of complex calculations and by the end of 12 weeks Annie's placement report specifically acknowledged her skills in drug administration and calculation.

In addition, to support her evidence for 'application of number' Annie presented a research assignment which utilised the gathering of statistical information, its presentation and analysis. Following a discussion with her mentor Annie decided these were the most appropriate forms of evidence to include in her key skills portfolio.

Employment and key skills

It has been argued by some that training and the world of work has undergone a major shift in emphasis over the past two decades. We have seen the development of competence and work-based training leading to qualifications such as National Vocational Qualifications (NVQs). We have also seen a shift in emphasis towards the employer taking responsibility for career development and management systems such as individual performance review growing in many areas. This changing world of work aims to produce a flexible workforce, able to adapt and change to market needs. There is an increasing expectation from employers that workers will be able to transfer skills from one role to another and be able to identify strengths, weaknesses and training needs (Hull *et al*, 2005)

The NHS has embraced much of this change including the development of NVQs for healthcare workers, and other competency based qualifications. There has been a focus on continuing professional development (CPD) for qualified nurses and an expansion of skills and extended roles. The development of nurse consultants and specialist nurses has added to the need for evidence of skills and knowledge and training to support this. The Department of Health (1999, 2000, 2001) has produced a number of reports supporting this shift. Lifelong learning has become a key concept within healthcare as an avenue to CPD, evidence-based care and ultimately better patient care (Department of Health, 2001).

At all levels key skills may be used to demonstrate the skills required across a range of roles and tasks within the healthcare context. As employers look for evidence of a flexible, adaptable worker with transferable skills it is the key skills that could provide the evidence for this.

Employability, key skills and the portfolio

Securing initial post-qualification employment

The portfolio, as a record of learning and achievements, is a useful tool when seeking employment. It can act as a showcase of what you have done for presentation at an interview and will verify your achievements in a written form. Currently pre-registration nursing students may present at interview having already achieved nationally determined competences and specific levels of academic qualification, ie. at postgraduate, undergraduate or diploma level. Their portfolio may be a huge unwieldy document that may or may not be looked at by the interview panel. Many nursing portfolios give evidence of the national competences required for pre-registration programmes and may not give the potential employer details of transferable skills, flexibility or demonstrate the adaptability of the candidate. Many nurses devalue the portfolio and struggle to see its worth beyond the requirements of their course or programme of study (Dolan *et al*, 2004).

A portfolio which clearly identifies the achievement of key skills can demonstrate a range of both transferable skills and a link between theory and practice components. It can provide the potential employer with validated evidence of those transferable essential skills. So how can the portfolio be used at interview?

You should view your portfolio as part of the process of selection. On your application form you may describe yourself as 'an effective communicator' but what does that mean and where is the evidence to support the claim. A reference may go some way to providing this evidence but you may also have evidence readily available in your portfolio, from group work undertaken on courses, presentations, work-based assessments, written reports, etc. Being able to demonstrate your skills at interview with verified evidence could be the route to a successful job application. However, arriving at an interview with a lever arch file marked portfolio and handing this over to the panel is not an effective way to demonstrate your abilities. Using your portfolio at interview should be managed by you and in congruence with the interview process. An example of a transcript from an effective interview can be seen below:

Interviewer: I can see from your application form that you state you have effective communication skills. Can you give specific examples of how you have demonstrated a range of communication skills in practice

Interviewee: During my last placement I was involved in working with the multi-disciplinary team and communicating with a range of professionals, I also wrote reports under supervision for the team meetings. My last placement report highlights both of those specific examples (hands interviewer this piece of evidence). The report also acknowledges my communication skills when working with patients and their relatives. In addition I have used my communication skills to undertake an assessed poster presentation. I received excellent feedback from the lecturer and have written feedback here if you would like to see it.

In this situation the interviewee was able to identify evidence drawn from her portfolio which highlighted communication as a key skill. A further example is included involving Annie who we heard about earlier in this chapter during her meeting with her mentor.

Interviewer: The unit you have applied for uses a ranges of complex medication regimes, what evidence do you have that you have developed skills in drug administration and calculation?

Interviewee (Annie): I have undertaken a classroom-based assessment on which I scored 92% but I also wanted to be sure that I could transfer this into the clinical setting so on my 'medical' placement I worked to a specific action plan with my mentor to utilise every opportunity for routine and non-routine supervised administration. I have my placement report and my score sheet for the classroom-based test here (hands the evidence to the panel). In addition I have developed a range of skills working with statistics and complex calculations during my research module and although this was not specifically related to drug calculations it has given me much more confidence in handling data of all kinds.

The evidence shown during this interview not only links theory and practice but also demonstrates a proactive relationship between Annie and her portfolio.

Many interviewers use scenario-based questions and again you can be prepared by not only stating how you would manage that scenario but also by focusing on problem solving as a key skill and how the development of that skill throughout your programme has led to you transferring this to the given scenario.

Continuing professional development

The portfolio has a crucial role to play in CPD. Much of the research however suggests that portfolios become merely files of information, containing certificates of attendance on study days, with little reflection or focus. Literature also suggests that nurses find portfolios time-consuming and place little value on collecting evidence beyond the requirements of the professional bodies (Dolan *et al*, 2004). Using the key skills approach can provide not only a focus for the post-qualifying portfolio but also evidence for future employment or role changes. The portfolio in the post-qualifying period often needs to take a different shape as the evidence included may not be structured around a course, module or programme of study. The evidence may also need to be verified in different ways as its author may not be supervised on a daily basis.

In the post-qualifying period, identifying the key skills that are developing may be a more reflective process underpinned by courses and modules and also be based around roles undertaken. The reflective process has been discussed elsewhere but it is useful to note here that reflection on the development of key skills will enhance the post-qualifying portfolio. Models of reflection are applicable to the development of communication skills, application of number, information technology, problem solving, working with others and improving own learning and performance. Working within a specific environment or taking on a new task, role or responsibility will offer the opportunity for reflection upon the development of those key skills. Using reflection within the portfolio can also support the development of skills in critical thinking and problem solving that are crucial to nursing.

Many roles concentrate on the use of key attributes rather than specific skills and developing a key skills portfolio can support your evidence towards these. You may look at a role description and be able to provide evidence for the practical skills required but how do you give evidence of the wider skills? In the past applicants have often relied upon a detailed reference or just a description of relevant skills at interview but tangible and verifiable evidence can lie within the portfolio and examples of evidence for each of the key skills can demonstrate flexibility, adaptability, self-motivation and ability to identify learning needs.

In addition to the professional requirements of the PREP (Nursing and Midwifery Council, 2002) portfolio the current climate of identifying competence for specific roles, for example using the Knowledge and Skills Framework (KSF) and the implementation of Agenda for Change means that a 'live' portfolio is crucial to successful career development. McLean *et al* (2005) describe the development of a critical care portfolio linked to the NHS KSF competencies highlighting the potential for evidence of development across levels. This type of portfolio may be a development for the future for qualified nurses seeking to provide evidence of their competence against the KSF. The portfolio that tracks evidence not only for specific competences but also for key transferable skills will embrace the notions of lifelong learning and specific role competence. Below is an example of an individual who applied for a role change and wanted to take on a higher level of responsibility.

Interviewer: You have been in your current role for the past three years. What skills would you use to develop yourself in this new role?

Interviewee: I have looked at the role description and identified within my portfolio those essential areas where I already have skills that can be demonstrated. One of these areas is around the development of communication strategies. This was something that was undertaken in my current role using a specific approach and this worked well. I have a critical reflection of this in my portfolio. For the future I would use this approach to create a communication strategy within my new role.

For those areas of the role description that are 'desirable' and where I feel I need to develop my skills, for example, using the computerised database system, I would plan an approach with my line manager using action plans to ensure that I developed these skills. I feel that I would also be demonstrating key skills in problem solving and improving my own learning.

This approach highlights the ways in which the key skills can be seen as those transferable skills but also examining the portfolio prior to interview against the role description demonstrates a proactive approach to the interview.

Using a key skills based portfolio is one model of portfolio development and may include a degree of self-assessment of key skills or at least an assessment of which skills have been used to generate the evidence contained within the

Name of key skill	Evidence	Page/reference
Communication		
Application of number		
Information technology		
Improving own learning		
Working with others		
Problem solving		

Figure 5.1. Example of key skill evidence index sheet.

portfolio. The process of putting the portfolio together develops a range of skills in itself. Using the key skills model could enhance employability as it focuses the evidence on those key transferable skills employers are seeking.

It is possible to create a key skills theme through your portfolio should you choose to, with simple index pages being used to highlight where the evidence for each key skill exists. An example of this is shown in *Figure 5.1*.

Summary

In order to utilise key skills as a framework within your portfolio you need to be aware of how they are developing within it. This chapter has focused on introducing you to those transferable key skills as one model of portfolio development. The portfolio model you use may be laid down by the course you are undertaking or you may feel more comfortable following a familiar structure.

If you choose not to focus your portfolio around key skills it is useful just to have an understanding and awareness of them, as they are skills that you can take into any area of your working life, in nursing, when considering a career change or into your life outside of work.

References

Benner P (1984) *From Novice to Expert*. Addison-Wesley, California

Department for Education and Skills National Statistics1995 From: http://www.dfes.gov.uk/rsgateway/DB/SFR/s000573/index.shtml [Accessed 4 January 2007]

Department of Health (1999) *Continuing Professional Development: Quality in the New NHS*. The Stationary Office, London

Department of Health (2000) *The NHS Plan: A plan for Investment, a Plan for Reform*. The Stationary Office, London

Department of Health (2001) *Working Together, Learning Together: A Framework for Lifelong Learning in the NHS*. The Stationary Office, London.

Dolan G; Fairbairn G, Harris S (2004) Is our student portfolio valued? *Nurse Education Today* **24**: 4–13

Hull C, Redfern L, Shuttleworth A (2005) *Profiles and Portfolios: A Guide for Health and Social Care* (2nd edn) Palgrave Macmillan, UK

Jukes L, Gilchrist M (2006) Concerns about numeracy skills of nursing students. *Nurse Education in Practice* **6**(4): 192–8

McLean C, Monger E, Lally I (2005) Assessment of practice using the National Health Service Knowledge and Skills Framework. *British Association of Critical Care Nurses, Nursing in Critical Care* **10**(3): 136–42

Nursing and Midwifery Council (2002) *The PREP Handbook*. NMC, London

Nursing and Midwifery Council (2004) *Standards of Proficiency for Pre-registration Nursing Education*. NMC, London

Qualifications and Curriculum Authority (2004) *The Key Skills Qualifications Standards and Guidance*. QCA, London

Redman W (1994) *Portfolios for Development – A Guide for Trainers and Managers*. Kogan Page, London

Schon D (1983) *The Reflective Practitioner*. Basic Books, New York

CHAPTER 6

Continuing professional development and lifelong learning

Claire Bethell and Rosemary Shepherd

Introduction

Being in the right place, with the right knowledge and skills, at the right time and to be able to seize the opportunity to change your career direction; gain promotion; or move through a knowledge and skills gateway is an essential part of portfolio development.

This chapter sets out the political and organisational context of continuing professional development (CPD) requirements for healthcare professionals and the place of the portfolio as a means of recording all learning that takes place throughout a professional career. It goes on to explore the skills and attitudes necessary for successful CPD and lifelong learning and the maintenance of a professional portfolio. The portfolio as a means of recording and guiding all CPD activities is discussed, with a section on using the portfolio or profile of achievement as a means of gaining academic credit for professional development, through accreditation of prior learning (or experiential learning) that will provide progression towards a formal award. It sets out ways of using a portfolio to plan and resource CPD, with frameworks and exercises or activities to help you achieve this successfully.

The context of CPD

CPD is part of every healthcare practitioner's professional life. Frequently reflecting on practice, considering new knowledge and skills to be acquired and setting action plans to acquire them is part of being a professional practitioner and registrant of a professional body. But it has not always been so. While many healthcare professionals worked hard to keep up to date and gain new knowledge and skills, there was no requirement to do so until the late 1980s when professional and political measures were put in place to ensure CPD would become an essential part of remaining on the professional register for nurses, midwives and health visitors, with other healthcare professions following suit.

The political context

In 2001, Alan Milburn (then Secretary of State for Health) wrote that lifelong learning is about growth and opportunity, about making sure that NHS staff can acquire new knowledge and skills in order to realise their potential and to help shape and change things for the better. He suggested that lifelong learning is inextricably linked with the wider agenda for building, rewarding and supporting the NHS workforce for the future (Department of Health, 2001).

The aim of the government was to ensure that the NHS had a highly skilled workforce that was attracted to the service and the service was able to retain its skilled staff. The government's document *Working Together – Learning Together: A Framework for Lifelong Learning for the NHS* (Department of Health, 2001: iii) set out, for the first time, 'a vision and a comprehensive strategy for lifelong learning' for staff working in the NHS in England and developed the detail proposed in the NHS Plan (Department of Health, 2000). The document goes on to state that lifelong learning is about ensuring NHS staff are 'equipped with the skills and knowledge to work flexibly in support of patients and are supported to grow, develop and realise their potential'. The government sees lifelong learning as the key to delivering their patient-centred services. They suggested that traditional professional boundaries would become blurred, as skills and knowledge would be developed around the needs of the patient, rather than being part of the role of the practitioner.

Developments for nurses and midwives came with the improved working week for medical practitioners. Nurses were enabled to gain more advanced skills and this is continuing to grow. The NHS Plan also set the pace for more skilled services provided closer to patients' homes. The role of general practice nurses has developed beyond recognition over the past two decades, as general practices provide more skilled diagnostic services, management of long-term conditions and increasingly, minor surgical procedures. Supporting roles for healthcare practitioners in general practice surgeries and health centres have undergone a steady move from acute to primary care settings, with acute services providing outreach services into local communities. This has meant hospital services providing care for very sick, highly dependent patients, with many wards providing care that, in the past, would have been provided in intensive care or high dependency units. Ward-based staff have had to gain new knowledge and skills to care for their much sicker patients, while primary care nurses have also had to gain new knowledge and skills to care for patients requiring more intensive, longer-term care in their own homes. The Chief Nursing Officer published a document on modernising nursing careers (Department of Health, 2006a), indicating ways in which healthcare will be developing in the future.

The professional context

The notion of CPD has been part of nursing, midwifery and health visiting culture for many years, for those practitioners who have wanted to 'move on and up' – gain promotion or move specialism. In order to move into different areas of practice, educational programmes had to be undertaken, for example, nursing to midwifery, midwifery to health visiting. However, prior to the publication of the United Kingdom Central Council's (UKCC) Post-registration Education and Practice (PREP) Project report (1990), planning, managing and recording CPD was somewhat ad hoc in nature.

Practitioners very often repeated learning, could not articulate how they had developed their professional practice and rarely had clear goals to remain fit for changing practice. Back then, prior to the 1990s, if you had chosen to remain in a specific area of healthcare, you were not required to engage in any professional development for many years, indeed, until retirement. Registration with the professional body was a once in a professional lifetime event. Now, the climate is changing, with a statutory requirement for nurses, midwives and specialist community public health nurses to sign to state they have undertaken some form of professional learning activity to remain eligible for re-registration with the Nursing and Midwifery Council (NMC) and fit for practice. This has been a statutory requirement since February 2002, following the enactment of the Nursing and Midwifery Order 2001.

In 1995, every registrant with the UKCC was sent a package of fact sheets outlining the requirements for registrants to achieve the standards for PREP (UKCC, 1995). There was a long transitional period for practitioners to take on the requirement to engage in learning activities or professional development, in order to remain proficient, skilled and knowledgeable practitioners. Now, as a registrant of the NMC, each practitioner is required to satisfy the Registrar that 'he is capable of safe and effective practice' (Point 9). The Nursing and Midwifery Order 2001 goes on to state (Point 10b) that the practitioner must satisfy the Registrar that 'he has met any prescribed requirements for continuing professional development within the prescribed time'. While there is no mention of a portfolio or profile within the Order, the NMC does suggest that a profile of evidence is a way of describing the CPD undertaken by an individual registrant. In their booklet *The PREP Handbook* (NMC, 2006), the details are set out, with a clear description of the requirements and PREP standard and, on pages 10 and 11, a suggested proforma for recording your CPD experiences.

Following extensive review, the regulation of non-medical healthcare professions is being formalised by the Health Professions Council (Department of Health, 2006b) and as part of the regulatory processes, a system of CPD will be set out. With the broad generic framework of the Knowledge and Skills Framework (KSF) (Department of Health, 2004), there is, for the first time, a common language for shared competencies. Most NHS staff will have an e-record of their CPD activities and their link to the KSF. For those professionals working outside the NHS, maintaining a portfolio will enable them to plan, implement and evaluate the impact of their learning.

The organisational context

'Growing the NHS workforce so that we have the right number of staff, with the right skills, in the right place, at the right time' was the aim of Government in 2001 (Department of Health, 2001: iii). The Government goes on to state that the organisation has a responsibility to ensure that the staff it employs are able to provide a high quality of care, through appropriate education and skills development that are accessible and open. Part of this commitment is the development of individual staff member's personal development plans (PDPs), which will ensure that continuing professional development is matched to individual staff member's needs. The Agenda for Change structure and the KSF will ensure this is a more structured approach to CPD, with the needs of the organisation and the staff member being considered at the annual appraisal event. The government's document *Working Together - Learning Together* (Department of Health, 2001: 13) sets out the characteristics of a successful NHS learning organisation that attracts staff and retains them:

- A coherent, well-resourced learning strategy.
- Led strongly and consistently.
- Explicitly linked to the roles and skills needed to deliver local service improvements for patients and to the needs of staff.
- A system of appraisal and personal development planning for all staff, linked to organisational and individual needs, regularly reviewed.
- A demonstration that education and training, and access to learning and library resources, is available on an equitable, non-discriminatory and increasingly flexible basis to all staff groups.

Thus, organisations have a duty to ensure they provide the staff they employ with the resources necessary to remain fit for practice in an increasingly changeable service.

The aim of CPD

The key focus or aim of any CPD activity should lead to an improved healthcare service for users and should meet the organisation's needs (NHS Education for Scotland, 2003). It should ensure that patients and their families are able to benefit from a better qualified and motivated workforce (Deparment of

Health, 2001). For individual practitioners, their own aims for professional development should ensure that they have the right skills, at the right time, to provide the care they are employed to provide, but may also ensure they have the right skills to gain promotion or to move into a new area of practice. That, for some, means a two-pronged approach to their CPD, that may be of a longer term. Using a portfolio will help to plan appropriate goals for current safe practice, but also to gain new knowledge and skills to be ready and able to move to a new area of practice.

The principles of CPD

NHS Scotland (2003: 4) suggests CPD activities should:

* be centred on the knowledge and skills required by practitioners to enable them to provide a high quality service,
* be research, evidence and competency based,
* be directly relevant to improving patient/client health,
* lead to improving service delivery,
* be informed by national and international initiatives.

These principles certainly apply to formal, sometimes accredited, learning experiences, offered in-house or by external training/educational sources. They will relate directly to your organisation's needs or your own individual needs that you think will fit your organisation's needs now or in the future.

There may, however, be occasions when your CPD activity will be for your own personal development purposes, where it will have a direct influence on the activities you engage in out of healthcare work. For example, you may be a school governor of your child/children's school. In order to fully engage in the school governor work, you may need to attend some educational courses, undertake some reading, or shadow fellow, more experienced governors. Although you could not say it will directly improve patient care, you will be gaining transferable skills that you will take into your healthcare work. For example, you will gain communication skills working within a multidisciplinary team and negotiating for or raising funds. This experience and newly acquired skills will be utilised in some way within your healthcare practice. You may be engaged in all sorts of learning, for a wide variety of out-of-work experiences and you need to consider the knowledge and skills you are acquiring as a result. For example, I remember many years ago, a student nurse who was about to qualify and who was trying to develop her curriculum vitae, telling me she had no skills. On further questioning, she was a member of a rowing team and enjoyed embroidery as a pastime. I was able to point out that being a member of a rowing team required team-working skills that would be highly honed and that embroidery required excellent hand-eye co-ordination, essential for fine nursing procedures. You need to be able to consider what knowledge and skills you have or acquire in your out-of-work life, which can be transferred into your professional life.

So, to the above principles, I would like to add the following:

■ All your CPD (or continuing *personal* development) activities must be recorded in your personal professional portfolio.
■ You should be able to record the clear link between your learning and its application to your practice.

The skills and attitudes required

If you have no aspirations to move 'onwards and upwards', or you feel you do not need to acquire new knowledge to provide your current level of healthcare, then engaging in any sort of CPD activity requires a set of skills and attitudes. First and foremost is the skill of being insightful and reflective. Healthcare should be about more than just 'doing the job'. It should be about taking pride in the care you provide and constantly thinking about that care. It is important to remember that healthcare does not stand still. New research brings in new treatments, new drugs and new conditions. Patients are more knowledgeable and have access to much of the material that was once only available to professionals. If you think about the care you are now providing and compare it to the care you provided five years ago, you will realise that you have acquired new knowledge and skills.

Answer the questions in *Table 6.1* in order to help you draw up your own personal development plan.

What has this activity highlighted to you? Perhaps you have had a recent appraisal and this activity reinforced the personal development plan you and your appraiser drew up. Perhaps you are due to attend for your appraisal and this activity has raised some questions you would like to ask your appraiser, to assist in the development of your personal development plan.

In order to engage in CPD, you need to be motivated. It can be uncomfortable identifying a skills or knowledge deficit, recognising that you need to gain a new skill or more knowledge about an aspect of your care. Even self-directed study means taking time out of other activities in order to engage in a learning experience. Sometimes, you will be in a position to be supported by your employer to undertake a learning experience, with time allocated and fees paid, other times, you will have to self-fund, or find the time from your days off. However, your CPD might not need to take a long time. You might be able to address immediate learning needs quite quickly and within your own work time. It may be that your longer-term learning needs may need some time

Table 6.1. Framework to support action plan development

1. Where am I now and what am I doing? (write a statement)
2. What skills and knowledge do I have that support me in my job today?
    *   Special skills/knowledge relating to my discipline/specialty (list at least 3)
    *   Additional skills/knowledge that support learners in my workplace (list at least 3)
    *   Additional skills/knowledge that help me manage:
        myself
        my workload
        my team
        the unit/ward/department
3. Where is my specialty going in the future? If I stay in my present post and grade/band, what new skills/knowledge will I need? List at least three new skills or knowledge (these may be clinical, management, educational, research, quality, for example)
4. How will I gain the skills/knowledge I need in answer to Question 3?
    *   Formal courses? If so, what?
    *   Study days, conferences or personal study?
    *   Shadowing other experts, visits to other units, etc.
    *   Other means (list)
5. What is my time frame – when will I need these skills/knowledge – beforehand or as the skills become necessary? (list in number of months or years)
6. Who will help me gain these skills? (eg. manager, colleague, family, myself, the university)
7. Where do I see myself in 1, 3, 5 or 10 years time? (Why is this? Give 5 reasons)
    Sometimes, there is a long-term goal, but there are intermediate steps along the way, with 2–3 years consolidation and acquisition of knowledge and skills.
8. How will I get there?
    *   Is there a course that I need to take?
    *   Will it be through promotion?
    *   Will it be through the unit/trust restructuring?
    *   Other reasons?
9. Who will help me get there?
10. What is my preferred time frame?
    If I cannot achieve that time frame, what will I do mean time?
    Think – will I be in the right place, at the right time, with right skills, to seize the opportunity?

commitment. Read through the critical incident analysis in *Table 6.2*, and try to relate it to your own recent reflective accounts.

From this activity, you can see the cyclical nature of reflection on practice, that there are short-term, medium-term and longer-term commitments. In addition, this sort of critical analysis considers the responsibility we all have, as registrants of a professional body and of sharing our expertise with others. The NMC (2004 clause 6, pp 9–10) Code of Professional Conduct, (mirrored by the Department of Health, 2006a) states that 'as a registered nurse, midwife or specialist community public health nurse, you must maintain your professional knowledge and competence'. There are five points to this clause, related to your own professional obligations to remain up-to-date, to practise competently, to seek help and supervision when working beyond your competence, to facilitate the development of skills and knowledge among learners and others to enable them to develop their competence, and to deliver care based on current evidence, best practice and research. So, what all this is saying, is that to act as a professional healthcare practitioner, you must continue with your professional development.

The professional portfolio as a guide to CPD activities

The NMC (2004, 2006) gives clear guidance on the need for CPD and see registrants as the individuals who are best placed to identify their own learning needs in light of their current practice. The portfolio is the tool that will enable registrants to identify through self-assessment constructive learning plans, which are achievable and will meet their personal and professional requirements. It will also be the tool that gives structure to the recording of learning and for the planning of further learning. One of the advantages of the professional portfolio is that it allows for the unexpected, or the serendipitous learning that takes place in the course of a registrant's career, to be recorded. It enables this learning to be developed and, where appropriate, plans for dissemination of such learning to be constructed and in turn recorded. The well-constructed and used portfolio will be registrants' record of their unique development and contribution to their profession. It will allow for individuals to prove their right to practice within their profession as it will be evidence of maintaining professional knowledge and competence (NMC, 2004) and to practice safely, effectively and legally within their evolving scope of practice (HPC, 2006).

The majority of registrants have to balance the demands of a busy professional life with the multiple roles and obligations they have in their personal lives (Weedle *et al*, 2002). For many individuals these are intertwined and the thought of structuring their CPD activities and maintaining a professional portfolio can, at times, seem like running a marathon, challenging and never ending. There are many benefits to creating and developing a

Table 6.2. Critical incident analysis

Alison, a specialist community public health nurse, visited a family new to her caseload. The family had recently moved into the area, with their 2-month-old son John, who was born at 38 weeks gestation and had experienced some difficulties in the peri-natal period. Further investigations that are still on-going are suggestive of ... syndrome.

Alison has not heard of this syndrome and feels uncomfortable that she cannot answer John's parents' questions. Alison knows that she is professionally responsible to act on her feelings (Nursing and Midwifery Council, 2004).

Stage 1: The reflective analysis
- What is it?
- What do I know?
- What do I not know?

Stage 2: Planning my immediate CPD
- How will I find out what I do not know?

Stage 3: Taking action
- Undertaking a literature review
- Contacting the ... self-help group
- Liaising with John's consultant and GP

Stage 4: Further reflection
- What more do I need to know?
- What are my new knowledge deficits?
- What are my new skills deficits?

Stage 5: Planning my longer term CPD
- How will I address these deficits?
- What is my personal development plan?

Stage 6: Sharing with others
- Who else needs to know?
- How will I disseminate my new knowledge and skills to those who need to know?

Stage 6: Practice development
- Are there practice developments that arise from my critical analysis and action plan?
- What are they?
- How will I be able to lead those developments?

portfolio and the degree of personal achievement can be immense. Careful assessment and planning of CPD activities is necessary to ensure that they meet personal, professional and institutional or employer needs. Registrants may ask the following questions.

How do I find time for this?

To find an answer it may be useful to take a holistic approach to your life and explore the roles you undertake. These roles may fall into two board categories: professional and personal.

It would be useful at this stage to take a few minutes to consider the roles that you carry out and how these roles make demands on your time. Ensure that you include the roles that you do for pleasure as well as the ones that you undertake from necessity; it is important to have a balanced approach to this activity to allow for honest acknowledgement of the time given to all aspects of life. This may help develop some clarity and context in which to plan time for appropriate developmental activities.

Having identified that time is a precious resource that needs to be used effectively the next question may be:

Where do I start?

Opportunities for annual appraisal or individual performance review may be a catalyst for self-assessment, the first stage of effective planning for CPD. An initial action may be to undertake a review of your current position. Undertaking a short piece of autobiographical writing could do this, exploring where you are professionally, what your skills are and where you see there are gaps in your knowledge and skills, or through a SWOT (strengths, weaknesses, opportunities, threats) analysis. The principles of SWOT analysis are shown in *Table 6.3* and the process is also referred to in *Chapter 2* where an example of a completed SWOT analysis is included.

Effective self-assessment requires not only acknowledgement of one's abilities, it also demands that areas of expertise should be supported by evidence of achievement. For instance, if you consider that you have an ability to communicate effectively with others, then some evidence of this should be available to support the statement. This could be in the form of feedback received from peers, managers or clients, invitations to contribute to team meetings where communication skills form part of the agenda or evaluations following presentations. It could also be supported by reflective practice, how an aspect of communication that may or may not have demonstrated good practice was explored and analysed and how this influenced future practice, perhaps including how this was disseminated to others.

Table 6.3. A SWOT analysis process

Strengths	*Weaknesses*
• What do you do well?	• What could you do better?
• What is unique about you?	• What do you lack in the way of
• What do others identify as	knowledge and/or skills?
your strengths?	• What do others see as your
	weaknesses?
Opportunities	*Threats*
• What professional opportunities	• Are there professional challenges
are open to you?	that put you in a vulnerable
• What professional trends do you	position?
wish to take advantage of?	• Are there situations that you find
• How can you use your strengths	competitive?
to support the opportunities	• What threats do your
available?	weaknesses expose you to?

Weakness or limitations should be addressed in the same manner. Consider the evidence that indicates a weakness. Why do you consider this to be a weakness and how can this be turned into a strength, what resources do you need to achieve this, are they available and realistic and will addressing this weakness/limitation benefit you, your practice and your employer?

Undertaking a SWOT analysis may enable exploration of the current trends in healthcare; this may feature in the opportunities section. Looking at the knowledge and skills that you possess and use in your current practice may help you to identify gaps in your repertoire – sometimes expressed as weaknesses or limitations – that could be addressed through specific learning activities.

Threats should not be ignored; they should be given as much detailed thought as the other aspects. Again put the threats you identify into context by providing evidence to support the premise that they are threats and then consider how they could be turned into opportunities. As part of this self-assessment it may also be useful to review how you learn, what strategies suit you best. Knowing how you learn may enable time to be used effectively; there are different ways of assessing your learning style, for instance the Honey and Mumford Learning Styles Inventory or the Myers Briggs Type Indicators.

Having undertaken some form of self-assessment the next step will be planning the CPD activities that will meet the gaps or developmental needs identified.

For the majority of registrants there will be a need to undertake some form of goal or objective setting once gaps in knowledge and/or skills that need to be addressed to enable professional development have been identified. This may be an activity that the individual can control. However, it may be necessary to negotiate with others, for instance employers where there are funding and/or study time release or institutional implications. The registrant may wish to explore opportunities for sponsorship within their employing organisation or from scholarships and bursaries available through other organisations. There are many CPD activities that may be achieved through day-to-day practice and work-based learning that do not require specific funding.

Consider the resources available. They may include:

- *Workplace*: If you are in employment, self-employed, or a voluntary worker one of the most influential learning environments is your workplace. Take time to explore the learning opportunities that occur on a daily basis. Does your employer provide you with in-house training, for instance to meet mandatory requirements such as resuscitation or emergency drills?
- *Peers*: Exploring issues with your peers may allow you to develop a wider perspective on practice and current influences in practice. Does your practice area encourage discussion related to day-to-day issues, is there opportunity for reflection with others, are there debriefing sessions following critical incidents?
- *Clinical supervision*: Is there a planned programme of clinical supervision in the area in which you work, is it possible to organise an appropriate clinical supervisor and are you able to negotiate time to spend in supervision sessions?
- *Specialist practitioners*: Do you meet specialist practitioners in your practice area, have you an understanding of their role, is it possible to arrange time with them to observe their practice and discuss their role?
- *Multidisciplinary team*: Do you meet with other healthcare practitioners, does your area hold team meetings, do you attend these, are there other meetings that relate to your practice that you could attend?
- *Libraries*: Does your employer have a library, have you access through your employment to an online library, do you have access to the local university library?
- *Internet/intranet facilities*: Do you have the skills to use a computer, are you comfortable using search engines, are these available to you at work, do you have access to the web at home or through your local library?
- *Policies and procedures*: Are there up-to-date, evidenced-based policies and procedures in you workplace, do you refer to them?
- *Professional organisations*: Do you belong to a professional organisation, do you read the literature they send, do they hold information sessions or conferences, are you able to attend these, do you undertake an active role in your professional organisation?

Thought should be given to the approach that is taken to the planning of goals or objectives and the individual needs to be clear if this is a long-term goal or objective that is a vision of the future, for instance:

In five years I will be working as a modern matron in a primary care setting.

The registrant is setting the long-term goal that has effectively developed a framework on which to base short-term goals that contribute to the vision for the future, therefore short-term goals could be:

In my role as a staff nurse in a primary care setting I will develop the skills required to assess clients' ability to comply with medication regimes, I will ask my preceptor to assess my ability to do this within the next year.

As part of my undergraduate studies I will undertake a literature review that will explore the efficacy of the role of modern matrons, this will be completed within the next two years.

The first goal could be achieved through day-to-day observation of practice, recorded in a reflective diary and further developed through reflective writing. Observation and discussion with the preceptor would confirm ability or allow for further formative work to be undertaken. To achieve the second goal the registrant may have to negotiate some sponsorship for his or her studies in the terms of support with fees and/or time release from the practice area.

There will be several short-term goals or objectives that will need to be achieved to fulfil the long-term vision. All the goals or objectives should be clearly written, using the acronym SMART which will help develop specific statements that effectively guide activities. SMART stands for:

- *Specific*: Is the statement clear and well defined, does it clearly state what needs to be done?
- *Measurable*: Does the statement clearly state what and when things need to be done?
- *Achievable or appropriate*: Do the resources exist for the goal to be achieved, is everything in place, is there value in this individual undertaking this development?
- *Relevant or realistic*: Does this fit with the current professional climate, is there a clear benefit in undertaking this development?
- *Timely*: Does the statement include the timeframe for achievement, is this realistic?

The principles of SMART are discussed in detail in *Chapter 2*.

January	February	March	April	May	June
Literature search					
	Review literature	Write notes and establish themes Additional search			
			Refine notes		
				Write review	
					Proofread review

Figure 6.1. Gantt chart used for planning a literature review.

Once the self-assessment has taken place and the objective or goal setting has happened it is then necessary to undertake some action planning. This can be a simple list that indicates the tasks to be undertaken and the timeframe in which they should be done or it could be in the form of a Gantt chart (see *Figure 6.1*).

As with any project it is useful to return to the plan on a regular basis. This will enable a review of progress and allow identification of where, when and how the next activity should be undertaken. Regular review will also help identify unrealistic goals and/or timeframes; it may also help identify what resources are required and when support should be sought.

Once any continuing developmental activity has been undertaken it is essential that some form of evaluation of the learning takes place. For the short-term goals that have already been stated evaluation is identified, for the first goal this is through observation and discussion, for the second goal this will be through achievement of academic outcomes. Evaluation of the learning should form part of the professional portfolio. As registrants become more comfortable with the portfolio they may find that the initial evaluation of a learning activity leads to further reflection, and, through this, identification of future learning activities. This reflects an active approach to CPD and lifelong learning.

Not all CPD activities undertaken will be planned in a formal manner, much of the learning undertaken will be serendipitous; it will happen as a result of the registrants' day-to-day practice. Kate's story illustrates how it is possible to use a short incident to show professional development.

> Kate arrived on duty to find that she had a pre-registration student, Amy, allocated to her for the shift. Amy seemed to avoid making contact with one patient who was about to have a minor investigation carried out under general anaesthetic. Kate decided to discuss the patient's care needs with Amy drawing attention to the psychological and physical care that the patient required. Amy expressed surprise that the patient should be so anxious over 'something minor'. Following a discussion Kate directed Amy to some of the literature held in the resource file about patient anxiety, agreeing to meet following day to share information and look at evidence to support best practice. Kate decided to review the support she had given the student, thinking that she may have contributed to the student's perception by the way in which she had given information to Amy. Following discussion with her supervisor and a peer Kate undertook a brief literature review about nurse perceptions of anxious patients to prepare herself for the planned meeting with Amy. Kate recorded this in her reflective diary and later extended the reflection through structured writing. She took this experience to the next mentors' meeting as a focus for discussion on student support. All of these activities featured in her professional portfolio.

In undertaking this activity Kate was able to demonstrate that her knowledge was up to date, that she was willing and able to facilitate Amy develop knowledge and skills based on best current evidence, practice and research and, through actively seeking supervision from her peers and fellow mentors, that she was willing to develop her own knowledge and skills. She was demonstrating her ability to practice as a competent registrant (NMC, 2004).

Using the personal and professional portfolio to claim credit for prior learning

The dynamic nature of healthcare with its demands for the safe and effective delivery of care, requires all practitioners to keep up to date with developing knowledge and technology and to demonstrate this currency of knowledge, technical skills and competencies within their day-to-day practice. This requires practitioners to undertake active learning, much of which occurs in the workplace, through in-service training or in a serendipitous manner. This is congruent with the demands professional bodies make on registrants who are required to ensure that their practice is safe, effective and meets the legal requirements of the country in which the practice is undertaken (NMC, 2004; Health Professions Council, 2005). This professional updating activity is monitored through the professional portfolio or profile of the individual practitioner. Frequently there is no formal recognition of this learning.

Accreditation of prior learning is a means of offering formal recognition of knowledge, skills and competency that have been acquired through experiential and/or formal learning. In short it places a value on previous learning, reflecting the political and professional agenda to recognise lifelong learning.

This is a process that may be useful to consider when identifying the next stage of your formal learning. Accreditation of prior (experiential) learning (AP(E)L) may offer you access to a course of study through proving your ability to demonstrate a specified level of academic ability or it may enable you to demonstrate that you have already met specified learning outcomes through pervious experiences. When considering AP(E)L it is important to remember that the process will demand demonstration of learning that is similar to undertaking a formal learning process and it will be measured against criteria that reflect academic level and/or practice requirements. There will normally be a further requirement to demonstrate currency of knowledge, skill and/or competence and subsequently most higher education institutions will anticipate that the learning will have been undertaken recently, for instance in the past five years.

A systematic review of learning undertaken in the past five years may be a useful starting point. Consider writing your own professional development story, this will help to identify your strengths and limitations and answer the following questions

- What have I done that demonstrates learning?
- Has this learning contributed to a formal qualification?
- How can I provide evidence of this learning?
- Does this learning have currency?

Read Diane's story and identify aspects that may indicate learning that could form the basis of an AP(E)L claim.

I qualified as a registered nurse five years ago when I completed my training and the Diploma in Higher Education. Since then I have worked as a staff nurse on an oncology unit in a district general hospital. I have been very involved in a change of practice relating to meeting the care of patients needing help with oral hygiene. This all started when I cared for a patient who had halitosis and a very sore mouth with some ulceration. I did some structured reflection, something that was a chore as a student but has become more meaningful as I've developed specific interests. I used Gibbs' Cycle of Reflection and realised that the structure not only offered me the opportunity to explore oral hygiene and why some nurses sometimes do not consider it a high priority but also directed me to explore broader issues, ie. the detailed anatomy and physiology of the mouth and the effects of some cytotoxic drugs. As my interest developed I was asked to contribute to an audit on oral hygiene, which gave me the opportunity to discuss this aspect of care as well as to observe the care given. Following this I did a presentation to the unit staff on oral hygiene and where we were able to demonstrate good practice. I tried to present from the positive perspective and staff were able to identify where they could improve, this resulted in a policy change and further audit, which showed an improvement in care as there was a decrease in the number of patients with mouth ulcers. I still have the letters of thanks from the audit department and the ward manager. I'm pleased when other staff direct new staff and students to me for advice on this area of care.

The grid in *Table 6.4* shows the learning that Diane identified through her autobiographical writing, the currency of the learning and the evidence there was to support her work.

Diane found that the evidence fell into two categories, "hard" or direct evidence and "soft" or indirect evidence (see *Table 6.5*).

If Diane wished to submit this profile of learning taken from her professional portfolio as evidence to support an AP(E)L claim it would need to meet the specified criteria; it may prove her ability to undertake higher level study or it may be used for specific credits which will be mapped to specific learning outcomes. The evidence supporting the claim will need to be scrutinised to ensure that it meets the appropriate criteria. Academic staff who review the evidence may ask Diane to justify some parts of her claim, this discussion will usually be part of an informal meeting.

Collating evidence from your professional portfolio to support an AP(E)L claim is usually straightforward, provided the registrant keeps focused on the purpose of the claim. One of the pitfalls is the temptation to include everything within the professional portfolio. Always ask questions about how something contributes to the claim, does it fulfil the stated outcomes or prove an academic level? All higher education institutions will have someone who can advise on the AP(E)L and who will be able to give guidance on compiling a claim.

Summary

Continuing professional development and lifelong learning complement each other, one will not occur without the other and both are essential elements of a dynamic learning organisation that needs to respond to the local, national and international healthcare agenda. Opportunities for learning and development are available to all registrants in day-to-day practice as well as through planned formal learning events. Individual registrants have a professional responsibility to demonstrate their right to practice through the recording of their own learning. The use of a professional portfolio will allow registrants to demonstrate their professional development through accurate records of learning events, planned

Table 6.4. Grid showing identified learning

Date	Learning activity	Evidence of learning
3 years ago	Reflection on mouth care, exploration of evidence base	Reflective writing using a structured model
3 years ago	Anatomy and physiology of the mouth Complied resource folder on evidenced-based oral hygiene	Notes on work, resource folder, copy of presentation to staff
3 years ago	Drugs, effects and side-effects	Notes on work undertaken, diary note of time spent with pharmacist
2 years ago	Participated in audit of patients' hygiene needs with specific emphasis on mouth care	Audit report, letter of thanks from audit team
2 years ago	Presentation to staff about audit findings and current evidence base for best practice	Presentation, handouts and paper to support presentation, letter of thanks from the ward manager
2 years ago	Worked with unit and clinical governance staff on new policy for mouth care	Minutes of meetings and current policy
1 year ago	Participated in audit of patients' hygiene needs with specific emphasis on oral hygiene	Audit report, letter of thanks from the audit team
9 months ago	Reported on audit findings to unit meeting, updated evidence-based material for unit file	Minutes of unit meeting, resource folder
Currently	Acting as a resource for new and established staff who wish to know more about mouth care in oncology	Part of day-to-day activities, difficult to evidence, I could consider asking unit manager and identified staff to write testimonials

Table 6.5. Categories of learning

Evidence of learning	Hard evidence	Soft evidence
Reflective writing using a structured model	This should demonstrate knowledge and understanding, it may also indicate the academic level of writing and ability to access evidence to support her work	
Anatomy and physiology – notes on work, resource folder, copy of presentation to staff	This should reflect knowledge base, and include detailed explanations and sources of reference	
Notes on work undertaken, letter of confirmation of meeting with pharmacist, copy of letter of thanks from Diane	The notes should reflect knowledge base	Letter acknowledging appointment confirms agreement to meet, letter of thanks indicates meeting took place
Audit report, letter of thanks from audit team	Audit report should acknowledge Diane's role in the audit	Letter confirms input
Presentation, handouts and paper to support presentation on oral hygiene, letter of thanks from the ward manager	This should include detailed explanations, diagrams and sources of reference	Letter of thanks confirms Diane undertook the presentation
Minutes of meetings and current policy		Indicates Diane's contribution to the work undertaken to develop the policy
Audit report, letter of thanks from the audit team	Audit report should acknowledge Diane's role in audit process	Letter of thanks confirms participation

Table continues

Table 6.5 continued

Evidence of learning	Hard evidence	Soft evidence
Minutes of unit meeting, resource folder	Provided they acknowledge Diane's contribution	
Part of day-to-day activities, difficult to evidence, could consider asking unit manager and identified staff to write testimonials		Testimonials would act as confirmation that this was part of Diane's role, it would also indicate her ability to support others' development

learning activities and developmental experiences. An up-to-date portfolio will reflect the registrants' ability to plan, record and assess their own learning and may be used to support future personal and professional development. It may also provide evidence that could support a claim for accreditation for prior learning and will support the registrants' right to remain on the professional register.

References

Department of Health (2006a) *Modernising Nursing Careers: Setting the Direction.* From: http://www.dh.gov.uk/cno [accessed 10 September 2006]

Department of Health (2006b) *The Regulation of the Non-medical Healthcare Professions: A Review by the Department of Health.* From: http://www.dh.gov.uk/publications [accessed 10 September 2006]

Department of Health (2004) *The NHS Knowledge and Skills Framework (NHS KSF) and the Development Review Process.* From: http://www.dh.gov.uk/PolicyAndGuidance/HumanResourcesAndTraining/Modernisingpay/AgendaforGaange/fs/en

Department of Health (2001) *Working Together – Learning Together: A Framework for Lifelong Learning for the NHS.* From: http://www.doh.gov.uk/lifelonglearning [accessed 12 December 2006]

Department of Health (2000) *The NHS Plan.* Department of Health, London

Health Professions Council (2006) *Continuing Professional Development and Your Registration.* From: http://hpc-uk.org [accessed 31 December 2006]

NHS Education for Scotland (2003) *Making Continuing Professional Development Work.* From: http://www.nes.scot.nhs.uk [accessed 14 July 2005]

Nursing and Midwifery Council (2006) *The PREP Handbook.* From: http://www.

nmc-uk.org [accessed 3 September 2006]

Nursing and Midwifery Council (2004) *The NMC Code of Professional Conduct: Standards for Conduct, Performance and Ethics*. Nursing and Midwifery Council, London

The Nursing and Midwifery Order 2001: Statutory Instrument 2002 No.253. From: http://www.opsi.gov.uk/si.si2002/20020253.htm [accessed 1 December 2006]

United Kingdom Central Council for Nursing, Midwifery and Health Visiting (1990) *The Report of the Post-registration Education and Practice Project*. UKCC, London

United Kingdom Central Council for Nursing, Midwifery and Health Visiting (1995) *PREP and You: Maintaining your Registration; Standards for Education Following Registration*. UKCC, London

Weedle DO, Himburg SP, Collins N, Lewis R (2002) American Diabetic Association. *J Amer Diabetic Assoc* **102**(10): 1439–548

Further reading

Challinor J, Wood R (2005) *Me and My PDR: Preparing for Your Personal Development Review (PDR)*. NHS Careers, London

Department of Health (2004) *Learning for Delivery: Making Connections between Post-qualification Learning/Continuing Professional Development and Service Planning*. Department of Health Publications, London

Department of Health (1999) *Continuing Professional Development: Quality in the new NHS*. http://tap.ccta.gov.uk/doh/coin4.nsf

Driscoll J, The B (2001) The contribution of portfolios and profiles to continuing professional development. *J Orthopaedic Nursing* **5**: 151–6

Furze G, Pearcey P (1999) Continuing education in nursing: A review of the literature *J Adv Nursing* **20**(2): 355–63

Nursing and Midwifery Council (2006) *A–Z Advice Sheet: Personal Professional Profiles*. http://www.nmc-uk.org

United Kingdom Central Council for Nursing, Midwifery and Health Visiting (1997) *PREP and You*. UKCC, London

CHAPTER 7

The portfolio as an empowering tool

James Dooher

Introduction

During the early 1990s portfolios became an fundamental part of a nurse's kitbag and, prompted by the UKCC (1990a, b; 1992; 1994; 1995), the process of completing and maintaining a professional profile or portfolio was deemed essential to demonstrate past achievements and future needs. Over a decade later, the emphasis on identifying, developing and releasing the talents of nurses continues to hold true.

This chapter explores the value of recording one's development as a part of reflective practice, enhancing the reader's ability to recognise, organise and showcase important elements of personal, academic, and career development. It will improve understanding of the need to maintain a qualitative self-centred and chronologically sequenced portfolio, providing concrete evidence of knowledge and experience to others, and at the same time enhancing confidence and self-efficacy for the portfolio writer.

Empowered nurses are able to celebrate their efforts, progress, and achievements from intra-, inter- and extra-personal perspectives. Empowered nurses are able to operate introspectively through reflection yet are also able to use their achievements as currency to demonstrate their wealth of experience, skill and knowledge. Investment in a portfolio enables nurses to demonstrate their past achievements and impress the portfolio reader with the notion that these can be replicated in future employment or education.

The concept of 'portfolios' or 'profiles' often means different things to different people but they are often a collection and interpretation of your work that allows your teacher, your employer (prospective or current) and other people to evaluate your abilities based on that work (Annis and Jones, 1995). In addition to the mandatory requirement for nurses to maintain a portfolio (UKCC, 1995), they serve as a record of personal development in which nurses can track their growth from both a personal and professional perspective. Portfolios provide evidence of your ongoing professional development accumulated over time, which exhibits the skills and abilities you possess. Portfolios could be considered as a reference book about yourself where career goals, samples of your work, your activities and accomplishments are recorded.

At the outset of a nursing career personal experience is a valuable commodity, but it is soon overtaken by the acquisition of professional experience and the knowledge base necessary to do the job in hand. Formal training, education and exposure to practice are all underpinned by personal experiences, both past and present, which run in parallel to the development of professional expertise.

As with the development of personal experience, professional experience is gained from learning and modelling, comprehension, testing and eventually mastery, or as Benner (1982, 1984) describes, the shift from novice to expert, becoming competent and proficient along the way. However, the process is not a linear one and often involves the reconsideration and review of knowledge or skill following mistakes. Errorless learning is a myth, and while making a mistake in one's personal life may be irritating, the consequences of a professional mistake may have serious and far reaching outcomes for one's career and, more importantly, the patients we serve. Accountability to oneself has been encouraged through the promotion of reflection in and on clinical practice, which capitalises on our innate desire to make sense of experiences and search for meaning. This in turn may help us learn from experience and become a more effective practitioner. When we utilise self-accountability with job-related accountability, our thoughts, feelings and behaviours are shaped into the actions, skills and outlook of a professional.

These elements of professionalism are seldom developed in isolation and often rely on an interdependent relationship with a mentor or, in the case of students, with a personal tutor. The development of a relationship with one's personal tutor adds real value to professional development.

Personal tutors are essentially the fulcrum upon which the theory/practice transfer is balanced, and a conduit through which the student may rehearse ideas and test values or understanding in a safe environment. The personal tutor can often make the difference between a student passing or failing to progress within a programme. They can motivate and confirm or reaffirm the content of a portfolio and assist in the development of coherent action plans which are realistic and achievable.

The empowering portfolio

Nurses who are empowered are better able to work productively and cooperatively (Dooher and Byrt, 2002). They possess and apply effective work habits and attitudes within the workplace and are able to work with others to complete tasks, solve problems, resolve conflicts, provide information, and offer support to their peers (Dooher and Byrt, 2003). Empowered nurses will value themselves positively, and apply principles of psychological wellness to their work and home life, being able to demarcate the two, and utilise processes such as clinical supervision to facilitate this. They will be able to articulate ideas more effectively and with confidence, and think critically and creatively applying the principles and strategies of purposeful, active, organised thinking. Empowered nurses will be able to learn from their mistakes and act responsibly to anticipate and prevent future mishaps.

One of the primary reasons that many nurses develop a professional portfolio or profile is as a response to Post-Registration Education and Practice (PREP) requirements when the availability of the profile becomes an essential part of the statutory periodic registration process. The consequences of failing to develop or maintain a portfolio may impact on one's ability to register or re-register with the Nursing and Midwifery Council, and it is the fear of these consequences that prompts many nurses to undertake this task. Behaviour that develops from fear can seldom be seen to be empowered behaviour, however we can draw solace from the fact that the substance and content of what is contained within it remains the choice of the portfolio writer. In addition, the style and layout of the work is also a matter of choice. This is underpinned by the plethora of templates available, some of which are developed locally and others nationally.

As with reflection, the strongest portfolios are often written for the writer as opposed to the reader, a notion that suggests that once the work is subject to external scrutiny it becomes contaminated (Dooher, 2001), losing the honesty and power of a private document. However, external assessment of one's portfolio provides the opportunity to enable others to acknowledge your growth and development. Often those involved in the assessment will focus upon its organisation, content and presentation, and it is this external assessment that provides the opportunity to nurture self-esteem and pride in one's work. The portfolio is a window into your ability to select appropriate examples of your experience and organise them in a way that is easy to read. The assessor can be assured of your writing skill and your ability to link concepts together and present them in a way that promotes your professional values. One might see the assessment process as a platform whereby your examples accentuate your skills, enhance the perception of your professionalism and provide proof of your plausibility. The positive image your profile creates may directly correlate to the success you achieve in sustaining employment or maintaining registration.

These factors are all well and good for those who have established a credible document but for those who are yet to start, or feel their profile is weak, the mandatory development of a portfolio may feel like a large stick with which they are about to be beaten. Such feelings are disempowering and often reduce motivation rather than galvanise the individual into action. However even these circumstances may lead to a positive outcome. Using the concept that 'it is the squeaky wheel that gets the oil', underperformance and failure to reach the required targets may result in additional support, training or other forms of help. In these circumstances your personal development plan or clinical supervision should highlight a need to secure assistance, and the organisation may feel obliged to enable you to access appropriate support. This strategy is inherently risky, but at the same time the need for staff development is recognised in most philosophical statements from organisations that place value on their human resource. Conversely, that same organisation may prefer to use your lack of evidence to initiate a performance management process whereby the absence of a portfolio is used as confirmation of limited development, and your failure to sustain professional knowledge or skill. In this scenario it is not the fact that you have failed to develop or eschewed opportunities, but a lack of the evidence that makes it difficult to prove what you have achieved, and how you have achieved it.

As far back as 1984 Benner recognised that embedded in the practices and the know-how of expert nurse clinicians there is a wealth of untapped knowledge, and she implied that this would remain dormant and unfertilised, never reaching its full potential unless it was systematically recorded. In turn, it is suggested that learning from one's own experience is enabled by recording and then reflecting upon the occurrences of professional life. If we assume this reasonably uncontentious statement is true, then we must acknowledge that the demands of the professional body (the Nursing and Midwifery Council) to record experience is a legitimate one which is appropriate and ultimately empowering.

Despite the good intentions of the NMC some nurses may well be overwhelmed by the notion of producing a record of their experience, and perhaps paralysed into inaction by the enormity of the task. However, in the same way one might advise a friend on the process of 'eating an elephant', small bite-size pieces are easier to chew. Goal setting is a simple way to sustain motivation establishing immediate, short-term, medium-term and longer-term objectives thereby breaking down the size of the task. In addition, ensuring one's expectations are realistic prevents over-reaching and the possibility of burnout. These goals should be realistic and achievable and, in order to have some end point, be set within a self-imposed appropriate timescale. When considering the commencement of the portfolio it is helpful to remember two key factors. Firstly the fact that 'today is the first day of the rest of your career' and as such recording today's activities for your portfolio is a portfolio, perhaps one that needs further development, but a portfolio none the less. The second point relates to perfection. Perfection is very difficult to achieve, and many of those who strive for it become disappointed and frustrated when they fail to meet their (or others') expectations. In this case the concept of 'good enough' is very useful in maintaining mastery over the process.

Dimensions of empowerment

The process of initiating and developing one's profile into a portfolio will promote a range of feelings within the nurse. The negative ones may relate to a resentment of the 'lost' time it takes to gather, organise and present the information. Undoubtedly there will be a cost in terms of time, although this will hopefully be outweighed by benefits of undertaking the exercise, and becoming an active participant in the review and development of one's career.

The range of benefits associated with improved control over one's career mirror the benefits of the empowerment process. Individuals' feelings of control and power over their destiny may well promote improvements in the following areas:

- skills, aptitudes and abilities,
- confidence,
- self-efficacy – belief in the capacity to bring about change,
- self-worth,
- pride in identity,
- the successful bringing about of desired change by the clinician,
- shifts, transfers or sharing of power from other professional groups or managers to the clinician.

Some definitions focus on only one of these dimensions. For example, empowerment has been defined as 'a process of helping people to assert control over the factors that affect their lives' (Fraher and Limpinnian, 1999: 146), and Braye (2000: 50) suggests that empowerment involves 'enabling people to acquire the skills and confidence needed to bring about improvements in the quality of their lives, or helping people to compete more effectively for scarce resources'. These definitions justify the notion that completing one's portfolio is a critical part of professional emancipation and the consequential empowering process that emerges.

Table 7.1 attempts to compartmentalise the elements of empowerment and illustrates some of the benefits of completing a portfolio that reflects on one's current professional circumstance.

The notion of empowerment has been conceived in many ways, but in this context is essentially seen as being that of active engagement enabling people to take control of their own career (Kendall, 1998). Taking control may be a slow process involving education and additional professional experience, together with support from peers and other colleagues and the person's range of social networks. Gibson described five stages towards empowerment which have been adapted to reflect the process a nurse may undergo during the construction of a portfolio. These are shown in *Table 7.2*.

Table 7.1. Elements of empowerment in portfolio construction

The belief in ability to have power, influence or control Professionals' willingness to share power/empower each other Individual's achievement of power or control over the organisation of care or wider service provision	Awareness of oppression (real or perceived). Negative feelings regarding professional authenticity Consciousness raising Pride in identity Increased self-esteem/self-image Increased internal locus of control Increased self-efficacy Inter-professional communication and relationships Professionals' facilitation of empowerment in: • Job satisfaction • Professional credibility • Securing new posts • Services provided Information Choice Consultation Having a voice Involvement in decision making

Table 7.2. Stages towards empowerment (adapted from Gibson 1995: 79)

Discovering reality including seeking information about the condition of career
Frustration related to limitations of education, resources and support from other professionals
Critical reflection in which the individual evaluates situations, develops confidence and takes positive action
Taking charge, including:
• Advocating for others
• Dealing effectively with systems
• Learning to persist
• Negotiation with professionals
• Establishing partnerships between differing professional groups
Holding on: the development of personal control, even in crises with the discovery of meaning and a sense of purpose

Enhancing confidence and improving leadership

Nurses often complain that having spent years developing their portfolio, the opportunities to share the information they have gathered with others are at best limited.

It is considered unusual for the Nursing and Midwifery Council to ask to see portfolios at the point of periodic re-registration and aside from perhaps clinical supervision, sharing one's development through a portfolio with others is a rarity. However, one platform upon which to celebrate your efforts is during a job interview. (Issues surrounding the interview process are covered extensively in *Chapter 5*.)

An increasing number of employers are requesting that candidates submit their portfolio as part of the selection process but anecdotal evidence suggests that these are still in the minority. It is therefore the candidate's decision to produce their work, and hope that it is taken into consideration. However, the actual value of the portfolio in an interview situation may be undermined by the constraints of the interview process itself. All too often a tight schedule of rolling interviews leaves those managing the process with very little time to explore the contents of a portfolio. In addition, interviewers are often surprised that a candidate is offering their work up for scrutiny, and their lack of experience underscores an inability to tell a good portfolio from a bad one.

All is not lost if your portfolio is ignored, because it is the process of collection and organisation of information that develops the confidence to respond to questions. This confidence is borne from a level of preparedness that indicates a formulated answer which has been considered over time, and rehearsed prior to the interview. As with exams, a period of revision prior to a testing situation will invariably improve self-confidence, self-belief and poise during the test. Without this process a prospective candidate may not be able to justify statements or refer to demonstrable evidence that sufficiently assures the panel. Ultimately those with a portfolio are more likely to get the job whether the panel look at the work or not

The maintenance of a portfolio enables authors to underpin for themselves, and demonstrate to others, an ability to function with responsibility, accountability and authority, which Øvretveit (1993) suggests are some of the key elements of leadership. Using your portfolio as a tool for developing others is a useful addendum to the skill set of a leader, and brings the work down from the dusty shelf, thus providing another opportunity to showcase your efforts. Developing an effective leadership style is often a challenging and complex process that demands a wide range of skills and personal characteristics. The notion of leading by example or modelling, is a useful way to create respect within a team, shape the thinking and behaviour of co-workers and instigate progressive change. When co-workers are given access to another's portfolio this will establish a milieu of transparency and honesty and enable the transformation from resistance and fear of portfolio development to one of acceptance and completion.

The concept of the transformational leader was coined by Burns (1978) who described this person as one who empowers, has a long-term focus and inspires through vision and ideals. Certainly sharing with others develops the possibility of empathy, and once this is achieved between co-workers cooperative opportunities improve and there is recognition of greater achievement, enhancing motivation and involvement in the leader's cause.

Some of the challenges facing the dissemination of good practice relate to the simplification and translation of what may be perceived as a complex process by the co-worker. It is useful to consider the work of Prochaska and Diclemente (1986) shown below, who provide a useful way of looking at change that helps the agent of change understand the process and difficulties which are likely to be faced.

- *Pre-contemplation*: Not considering the possibility of change, either because they are unaware of the need for change or unwilling to confront the problem.
- *Contemplation*: Aware of the existence of a problem. Seriously considering the possibility of change but feeling ambivalent. They see the benefits but feel distressed about the sacrifices involved.
- *Preparation:* Decided on their commitment to change and will make a change in the near future (within three months). Still some ambivalence.
- *Action*: Actually starting to make change in their behaviour. Might be confident in their ability to sustain change at the start.
- *Maintenance*: Attempting to sustain the progress achieved during action. Are likely to be constantly struggling with thoughts about relapsing. Lasts between six months and a lifetime.
- *Termination:* Free from the temptation to return to old behaviours. The new behaviour is more habitual than the old.
- *Relapse*: Not strictly a stage of change, but a possible outcome of action or maintenance. Unsuccessful in their attempt at change. Likely to go back into contemplation and seriously intend to make another attempt at change in the near future.

Encouraging others to commence and maintain their portfolio could be seen as beyond the call of duty, particularly when colleagues are professionally accountable for their own actions, and one must define the limits of intervention to encouragement and modelling. The final decision must rest with the individual staff member.

The following points should be considered when embarking on your portfolio journey and throughout the learning process:

- The power of your portfolio is contained in the process of its completion as much as the paper product or hard copy.
- If you have prepared a portfolio and it sits on a shelf gathering dust, or ignored during the interview process then it can lead in the short-term to deflated feelings, and in the long-term to a lack of motivation which ultimately undermines the essential value of portfolios in general.
- Completing a portfolio may raise self-esteem, increase pride in your professional identity, and improve inter-professional communication and relationships.
- Colleagues and co-workers must take responsibility for their own portfolios.
- Sharing a portfolio brings co-workers together in a mutual and common pursuit of a higher purpose, namely patient care and professional progression.

Summary

While the completion of a portfolio will not be a life-changing event in itself, it will facilitate the reflective process needed to instigate professional and personal change. It will reaffirm the individual's strengths and capabilities which in turn will promote a real sense of professional authenticity.

The net result of this will hopefully improve job satisfaction, professional credibility and the ability of individuals to secure the type of employment which best meets their needs and aspirations.

Nurses who have explored their strengths and weaknesses through the reflective element of a portfolio will have raised consciousness and be aware of what they do not know as well as what they do know. This understanding better enables the formulation of an action plan to remedy shortfalls in both knowledge and skill. It also helps shape understanding of professional and personal identity increasing self-esteem and self-image. The locus of control shifts from being externally orientated to internally orientated, which, by default, promotes self-efficacy.

It is pragmatic to anticipate that most interviewers will give portfolios scant attention, and to improve chances of success, candidates must try to distil their positive points into either their curriculum vitae, or the personal statement contained in the application form. This is where a well-organised portfolio is important, as discussed in *Chapter 4*. Only a proportion of the evidence gathered into the portfolio will form the basis of the application, and the candidate will need to be able to discriminate between ideas to find the most suitable pieces to match the post being sought.

References

Annis L, Jones C (1995). Student portfolios: Their objectives, development, and use. In P Seldin and Associates (eds) *Improving College Teaching* (p. 185). Ankar, Publishing, Bolton, MA

Benner P (1982) From novice to expert. *Amer J Nursing*. **March**: 402–7

Benner P (1984) *From Novice to Expert: Excellence and Power in Clinical Nursing Practice*. Addison Wesley, California

Braye S (2000) Participation and involvement in social care: An overview. In Kemshall H, Littlechild R. (eds) *User Involvement and Participation in Social Care*. Jessica Kingsley Publishers, London

Burns JM (1978) *Leadership*. (p. 224) Harper and Rowe, New York

Dooher J (2001) Reflections on reflection. In Dooher J, Clark A, Fowler J *Case Studies on Practice Development* (p. 158) Quay Books, Wiltshire.

Dooher J, Byrt R (2002) *Empowerment and Participation: Power Influence and Control in Contemporary Healthcare*. Quay Books, Wiltshire

Dooher J, Byrt R (2003) *Empowerment and Health Service User*. Quay Books, Wiltshire

Fraher A, Limpinman M (1999) Cited in Parry-Crooke, G. (2000) *Good Girls: Surviving the Secure System*. London. University of North London

Gibson CH (1995). The process of empowerment in mothers of chronically disabled children. *J Adv Nursing* **21**: 1201–10

Kendall S (1998) Introduction. In Kendall S (ed) *Health and Empowerment: Research and Practice*. Arnold, London

Prochaska J, DiClemente C (1986) Towards a comprehensive model of change. In Miller W, Heather N (eds) *Treating Addictive Behaviours: Processes of Change*. Plenum, New York

Prochaska J, Velicer WF, Rossi JS (1994) Stages of change and decisional balance for 12 problem behaviours. *Health Psychology* **13**(1): 39-46

Øvretveit J (1993) *Co-ordinating Community Care: Multidisciplinary Teams and Care Management*. Open University Press, Buckingham

UKCC (1990a) *Post-Registration and Practice, Project Discussion Paper*. UKCC, London

UKCC (1990b) *The Report of Post-Registration and Practice Project*. UKCC, London

UKCC (1992) *The Scope of Professional Practice*. UKCC, London

UKCC (1994) *The Future of Professionals: The Council's Standards for Education and Practice Following Registration*. UKCC, London

UKCC (1995) *PREP and You*. UKCC, London

Index